PRAISE FOR RICHARD
AND *THE SU*

D0645119

"*The Sugar Fix* stakes out new territory in the crowded field of dietary advice. But it is more than just another weight-reduction tutorial.... Dr. Rick Johnson and Tim Gower apply this knowledge skillfully in the design of a new and palatable way to reverse a long-standing obstacle to good health."

—Richard J. Glassock, MD,
professor emeritus of medicine,
David Geffen School of Medicine, UCLA

"Provocative, compelling, and a challenge to some of the classic paradigms."

—James O. Hill, PhD,
director of the Center for Human Nutrition,
University of Colorado Health Sciences Center

"Dr. Rick Johnson's new book provides compelling scientific evidence linking the current epidemic of obesity and diabetes with the progressive rise in fructose consumption, particularly over the last 30 to 40 years."

—Michael W. Rich, MD,
professor of medicine and director
of the Cardiac Rapid Evaluation Unit,
Washington University School of Medicine

"*The Sugar Fix* presents a combination of scientific research (the majority of it generated in Dr. Rick Johnson's laboratory), epidemiologic evidence, and historical insights, all linked together in the manner of a masterful closing argument before the jury retires for deliberation."

—Dr. Bernardo Rodríguez-Iturbe,
president-elect of the International Society
of Nephrology and international expert
on hypertension and kidney disease

THE SUGAR FIX

THE HIGH-FRUCTOSE FALLOUT THAT IS MAKING YOU FAT AND SICK

RICHARD J. JOHNSON, MD
WITH **TIMOTHY GOWER** AND
ELIZABETH GOLLUB, PhD, RD

Pocket Books
New York London Toronto Sydney

Pocket Books
A Division of Simon & Schuster, Inc.
1230 Avenue of the Americas
New York, NY 10020

First Pocket Books trade paperback edition May 2009

POCKET and colophon are registered trademarks of
Simon & Schuster, Inc.

For information about special discounts for bulk purchases,
please contact Simon & Schuster Special Sales at 1–800–456–6798 or
business@simonandschuster.com.

Manufactured in the United States of America

The Simon & Schuster Speakers Bureau can bring authors
to your live event. For more information or to book an event,
contact the Simon & Schuster Speakers Bureau at
1-866-248-3049 or visit our website at www.simonspeakers.com.

10   9   8   7   6   5   4   3   2   1

ISBN-13: 978–1–4391–0167–4
ISBN-10:   1–4391–0167–1

Notice

This book is intended as a reference volume only,
not as a medical manual. The information given here is designed
to help you make informed decisions about your health.
It is not intended as a substitute for any treatment that
may have been prescribed by your doctor. If you suspect that you
have a medical problem, we urge you to seek competent medical help.

Mention of specific companies, organizations, or authorities in this book
does not imply endorsement by the publisher, nor does mention of specific
companies, organizations, or authorities imply that they endorse this book.

Internet addresses and telephone numbers given in this book
were accurate at the time it went to press.

ACKNOWLEDGMENTS

I would like to give special thanks to writer Timothy Gower, who helped me to explain my research and ideas in lay terms; nutritionist Elizabeth Gollub, PhD, RD, who worked with me to construct the Low-Fructose Diet; and Chris Fennell, the superb chef and co-owner of the Northwest Grille in Gainesville, Florida, who provided many of the low-fructose recipes. I also want to thank Judith Riven, my agent, for helping to take this story from concept to bound book.

I have been fortunate enough to collaborate with many remarkable scientists. My sincere appreciation goes to Bernardo Rodriguez-Iturbe, MD, and Jaime Herrera-Acosta, MD, for our studies on high blood pressure; Marilda Mazzali, MD, Duk-Hee Kang, MD, L. Gabriel Sanchez-Lozada, PhD, and Daniel I. Feig, MD, for our studies on uric acid; and Taka Nakagawa, MD, Yuri Sautin, PhD, Sirirat Reungjui, MD, and Mark Segal, MD, for our work on fructose. I also remain forever indebted to Wei Mu, MD, and Carlos Roncal, BS, who oversee my laboratory and made significant contributions on all aspects of the research.

Finally, I would like to thank my wife and children for their patience and support, and my patients—it has been a privilege and pleasure to treat and care for you.

CONTENTS

PART IV   MORE THAN A DIET: THE LOW-FRUCTOSE LIFESTYLE

APPENDICES

INTRODUCTION

Dr. Chen's Observation

It had been a long day, but I was in the mood to celebrate. I had learned earlier in the week that an important scientific journal, the *Journal of Clinical Investigation (JCI)*, planned to publish a paper I had written based on my research. For a young scientist, this represented a major step toward gaining a full professorship at the University of Washington, where I worked at the time.

The future suddenly looked bright, so I accepted an invitation to a cocktail party at my boss's home. Soon after arriving at his lovely houseboat on Seattle's Lake Union, one of my colleagues, Dr. Yipu Chen, approached me. Yipu, a visiting scientist from Beijing, greeted me with his usual enthusiasm and said, "Rick, I believe you are going to be a professor some day. Yes, you will be a professor."

"Thanks," I responded, beaming with pride. I assumed that Yipu was about to compliment me on my *JCI* paper. I didn't want to seem presumptuous, however. So I asked, "Why do you think that?"

Yipu smiled. "Because you are getting fat, Rick," he said, patting my belly. "And in China, only the professors get fat."

I recalled this scene when I set out to write this book for

several reasons. For starters, I know what it's like to struggle with extra weight now and then. After Yipu made his good-natured jibe, I slipped away to the bathroom and looked in the mirror. He was right—I *had* put on a few pounds. Spending long days in the lab meant I wasn't getting enough exercise, and I was eating too much fast food. I vowed at that moment to make some important changes to get control over my weight problem.

Further, Yipu's comment says a great deal about what has happened globally over the past generation. This incident occurred more than 20 years ago, at a time when obesity was relatively rare in China and most other parts of the world. In Beijing of the day, only people with substantial incomes, such as university professors, could afford the luxury of eating too much.

Since then, though, China's economy has improved, and the people there, like people all over the world, have access to cheap processed foods that are high in calories, fat, and—significantly—added sweeteners. Not surprisingly, the world—not just the United States—finds itself gripped by an obesity epidemic.

How did we get to this point? And what can you do to protect yourself and counteract the effects of the modern diet? In this book, I will describe an all-new approach to weight loss and better health that is based in large part on cutting-edge research that I have conducted with my colleagues. We have identified a mechanism that makes your body ultrasensitive to sweet foods—a mechanism that I will show you how to turn off, helping you to maintain a healthy weight and safeguard yourself against many of today's leading disease threats.

As the title of this book suggests, I believe we need to

repair our unhealthy relationship with sugar. In the following pages, you will learn why consuming large amounts of one form of sugar in particular—known as fructose—can have devastating implications for your health. If the word *fructose* is new to you, rest assured that you are no stranger to this simple sugar. As its name implies, fructose gives fruit its sweet taste. It also binds together with another simple sugar, glucose, to form the white crystals you know as table sugar. Furthermore, fructose is the critical element in a commercial sweetener called high-fructose corn syrup (HFCS), which food processors add to a staggering array of products.

I wrote *The Sugar Fix* to inform and educate the public—and other doctors, too—about fructose's role in the current epidemic of obesity and its influence on rising rates of conditions such as heart disease, diabetes, kidney disease, and others. Week after week, studies appear in scientific journals offering evidence that a high-fructose diet leads to serious health problems. Yet even people who stay abreast of health news are probably aware of only a small amount of this research. For instance, you may have heard or read about studies linking soft drinks—a major source of fructose—to obesity. But we now know that consuming too much fructose can affect your overall health in many other ways, which I will discuss in the chapters to come.

My Path to Fructose

Though this book features a detailed diet plan that I will describe in Chapter 11, I never set out to discover a new approach to weight loss. Since early in my career as a scientist, I have devoted much of my attention to blood pressure. Specifically, my colleagues and I have been trying to learn what causes essential hypertension, the most common form of high blood pressure. Our research revealed that a compound called uric acid has an important influence on blood pressure. We subsequently learned that eating fructose stimulates production of uric acid. Before long, we realized that fructose was actually at the heart of an even broader health crisis. The data were alarming: Diets rich in this simple sugar appeared to be contributing to the growing obesity problem and rising rates of cardiovascular disease and other serious conditions.

As it became increasingly clear that eating too much fructose could make you gain weight and get sick, some people involved in our project began to experiment with their diets by cutting back on sugar, HFCS, and other sources of fructose. All of them lost a significant amount of weight.

One was Mike Guske, a 30-year-old hospital administrator. Mike's weight had risen to 205 pounds despite the fact that he's very active, playing soccer in a competitive city league three or four times a week. After he and I discussed his diet, it became obvious that he was consuming a great deal of fructose, largely from soft drinks and sugary foods. I instructed him to eliminate these foods and showed him how to identify other hidden sources of fructose. Within 6 weeks, he lost 20 pounds. As a bonus, his borderline-high blood pressure dropped by 10 points, which is the kind of reduction we would expect to see in a hypertensive patient who's given medication.

Word about the diet began to spread, and soon I was flooded with e-mails from people wanting more information about it. Which foods are high in fructose? Which are low? How can I tell on my own? To answer these questions,

I began to put together an early version of the plan that eventually became the Low-Fructose Diet. As I did so, I tailored the diet to limit intake of other food elements besides fructose that increase blood levels of uric acid, such as compounds called purines that are found in fatty meats, some types of seafood, and beer.

(I will include the stories of several other people who tried the Low-Fructose Diet and experienced substantial weight loss and other health improvements later on. In some cases, as noted, I have honored the privacy of these people by using pseudonyms.)

Uric Acid: The New Cholesterol?

Although the title of this book is *The Sugar Fix,* you will read a great deal about uric acid in these pages, too. As we are rapidly learning, fructose's effect on uric acid may explain why eating too much sugar is so unhealthy. In fact, I believe that we may one day discover that having high levels of uric acid in the blood could be as dangerous as having elevated cholesterol.

What we already know about uric acid is disturbing enough. My group has shown that increasing levels of this compound in laboratory animals cause their blood pressure to rise. A number of studies in humans have confirmed that people with elevated serum uric acid are at high risk for developing high blood pressure, even if they otherwise appear to be perfectly healthy. In another study, we evaluated teenagers who had recently been diagnosed with high blood pressure and found that nearly 90 percent had elevated levels of uric acid.

In 2007, we completed a very important study in which we gave obese children with hypertension two treatments:

First, the kids received a drug that lowers uric acid. Next, we gave them an "empty" pill (known as a placebo). In the first rigorously designed study of its kind, we showed that lowering uric acid levels in these children improved their blood pressure. Studies by other researchers suggest that lowering uric acid in adults with hypertension would produce similar benefits.

Because fructose causes uric acid to rise, it's no surprise that as consumption of sugary foods and beverages has increased in this country, so have typical blood levels of uric acid across the population. One recent study found that men who consume the most soft drinks also have the highest uric acid levels. I believe these trends help to explain why so many Americans are struggling with weight problems, elevated blood pressure, and other serious conditions.

I'm not the least surprised if you'd never heard of uric acid before opening this book. After all, most practicing physicians know little about it. Yet as of this writing, more than 3,500 articles have been published on the role of uric acid in human health, with more appearing in medical journals all the time. Nearly all of these studies to date show a strong relationship between uric acid and obesity, heart disease, hypertension, stroke, and kidney disease, among other conditions.

For example, Japanese researchers followed a group of men for 5 years and found that those with elevated uric acid gained four times as much weight as men with low uric acid. Likewise, studies consistently show that uric acid increases the risk for cardiovascular disease. In fact, some research suggests that having high uric acid doubles the risk for hypertension and increases the chances of dying from heart disease by four to five times. If your uric acid levels are silently setting the stage for serious health problems, there's a good chance you're consuming too much fructose.

The story of fructose and uric acid becomes more complex and layered every day, particularly as we learn more about how they cause obesity and cardiovascular disease. For instance, you may have heard or read about research in recent years suggesting that inflammation in the arteries triggers heart attacks. Some cardiologists now test for markers of inflammation to help predict which patients will develop cardiovascular disease. Yet no one has been able to explain why arteries become inflamed in some patients, but not others. Now we may have one important answer to this mystery. Our research has shown that even low concentrations of fructose can cause inflammation in vascular cells in the arteries. I will talk more about how fructose triggers inflammation and other risk factors for heart disease in later chapters.

The growing body of science on the harmful effects of fructose and uric acid has already begun to have an impact on society and health policy. As I mentioned earlier, studies have strongly linked fructose-rich soft drinks to obesity. Concerns raised by this research contributed to public pressure that encouraged the major producers of soft drinks in the United States to voluntarily stop selling their products in the nation's schools. Concerns about obesity have also led pediatricians to begin advising parents to limit their children's intake of fruit juice, which is also high in fructose.

The Low-Fructose Solution

As you read on, you will discover that the evidence against fructose and uric acid is quite compelling. That brings me to the good news I have to offer in this book: Making some simple dietary changes—by cutting back on fructose and a few other foods—can help you lose weight and reduce your risk for heart disease and other conditions related to metabolic syndrome.

The news gets even better. Research suggests that lowering intake of fructose can improve health in other ways as well. For example, high-fructose diets have been linked to liver and kidney disease, gastrointestinal disorders, short stature in children, eye disease, and even certain cancers.

What's more, cutting back on the amount of fructose in your diet will reduce your body's production of chemicals called advanced glycation end products. The acronym for these compounds—AGE—says it all: They appear to speed up the aging of cells, which may contribute to a number of chronic and fatal diseases. Gram for gram, fructose produces up to 10 times more AGEs than other common sugars in the diet.

If you have read other books that offer advice about controlling weight and improving health, what you have already absorbed in this introduction may come as a mild surprise, if not an outright shock. That's perfectly understandable. I believe that *The Sugar Fix* is the first book to expose and discuss this important health threat in any depth.

Furthermore, you may have read or been told that fructose is the "healthy" sugar, a less troublesome alternative to other sweeteners. In the past, for example, some doctors advised diabetes patients—who have problems controlling blood sugar—to sweeten food with pure fructose instead of refined sugar. The reason: Unlike other forms of sugar, fructose does not cause a dramatic rise in blood sugar.

Some patients still use fructose this way. I even know of one cookbook published some years ago that explains how to replace refined sugar in recipes with fructose.

Rest assured that you won't find much support for that particular cooking technique in the pages that follow. (To the contrary: I will present a variety of delicious low-fructose recipes in the appendix.) Throughout this book, you will learn that fructose has unusual metabolic qualities that truly set it apart from other types of sugar, rarely for the better.

Join the Low-Fructose Revolution

I am going to make specific recommendations that you can use to plan meals and decide how much fructose is safe to eat every day and which purine-rich foods you should avoid or limit. If you are like most Americans, you will need to make some significant changes to your diet, though I assure you that adopting a low-fructose meal plan is relatively painless—and unquestionably worth the effort.

Furthermore, I am going to recommend that you have your uric acid level measured from now on as part of routine physical exams. A uric acid assay is a cheap and simple analysis that any lab can perform when you have your blood lipids and blood sugar tested. In a later chapter, I will lay out goals to aim for as part of your overall health management plan.

Fair warning: Don't be surprised if your physician is skeptical when you ask him or her to measure your uric acid, or when you mention that you have adopted a low-fructose diet. I believe that these steps will help you to lose weight and safeguard your all-around health. In addition to the ongoing research in our labs, I have seen firsthand—in patients, friends, and colleagues—the health benefits of reducing fructose in the diet. I wrote *The Sugar Fix* with hopes that the millions of other Americans who continue to struggle with their weight could shed pounds and enjoy better health through the diet plan I have devised.

It's clear to me that we need a new approach to weight control, especially given the strain that excess body fat places on the human heart. Although modern medicine has made great strides in its ability to treat patients with cardiovascular disease, we need more weapons in our arsenal. Doctors can reroute the flow of blood past a clogged artery with coronary bypass surgery. As an alternative, vascular surgeons can use an angioplasty procedure to widen a narrowed blood vessel and then keep it propped open by inserting a fine mesh tube called a stent. Emergency room physicians have clot-busting thrombolytic drugs, which if delivered in time can literally stop a heart attack in progress.

Despite these incredible medical advances, cardiovascular disease mortality still accounts for 36 percent of all deaths in the United States. That's higher than the number of deaths in this country from cancer, accidents, and infectious diseases *combined*. I hope that the recommendations in this book will help to reverse the curse of cardiovascular disease, and at the same time help readers who follow the guidelines I spell out to achieve more immediate goals— namely, to lose weight, feel better about the way they look, and feel better—period.

While some of the information in this book will challenge, and even contradict, the theories promoted in other health and weight-loss guides, everything you are about to read is supported by a wealth of research published in top medical journals. The evidence linking fructose to today's epidemics of obesity, cardiovascular disease, and other medical conditions is as solid as the scientific data that connected smoking to lung cancer in the late 1950s and cholesterol to heart disease in the 1960s.

A bit of the information in these pages is somewhat technical, but I believe it's important for you to understand how shedding the fructose habit can pare inches from your waistline as it adds years to your life. With that in mind, I will do my best to make the science easy to understand and relevant.

In the interest of full disclosure, I would like to acknowledge that my colleagues and I have submitted several patent applications, from which I could benefit financially, based on scientific discoveries we have made related to fructose, uric acid, and cardiovascular disease. I want to assure you, however, that our research is completely objective and unbiased and meets the highest standards of science. Studies based on our findings have been published in top medical journals. That means they have passed "peer review," the process in which other scientists judge a study's quality and scientific integrity.

A lot of what you're about to read overturns long-held assumptions about fructose and uric acid, so I expect my message to meet with some resistance. I also believe that the theories you will read about in the pages that follow will one day be widely embraced by the medical community, though it may take time. After all, 50 years ago, the leading biochemistry textbook of the day stated that there was "no satisfactory evidence" that a high concentration of cholesterol causes heart disease.

Of course, scientists eventually proved that high choles-terol *does* increase the risk for heart attacks, which led to an entirely new way of thinking about the causes and pre-vention of cardiovascular disease. I believe that fructose and uric acid may be significant threats, too, and they loom larger every day. The historian Thomas Kuhn described sci-entific progress as a "series of peaceful interludes punctu-ated by intellectually violent revolutions," in which ". . . [o]ne conceptual world view is replaced by another." The Low-Fructose Diet is a new concept in weight loss and disease prevention. Welcome to the revolution.

PART I

CRYSTALS AND CORN SYRUP: A BRIEF HISTORY OF FRUCTOSE

CHAPTER 1

THE FRUCTOSE FACTOR

A Sugar Like No Other

A century ago, few Americans were overweight. Heart disease and diabetes were rare medical conditions. Today, people who are plump and paunchy outnumber those who are thin and fit in the United States and many other parts of the world. Heart attacks are the leading cause of death. The incidence of diabetes has exploded into a full-blown epidemic.

What happened? How could such dramatic changes to overall health occur during this relatively brief period in human history? I believe the rise of obesity and these formerly rare diseases can largely be traced to a single factor. Unlike a disease-carrying microbe, however, this culprit is hiding in plain sight—on the shelves at your local supermarket, in the cooler at the convenience store, and very likely in your refrigerator and kitchen cupboard.

The goal of this book is to help you understand, identify, and avoid this menace. What's more, I am going to show you how to reverse the damage it may have already caused in your system.

You don't need to be a doctor or scientist to see the most obvious signs of this scourge's handiwork. Simply walk through a shopping mall or playground—that is, if you haven't already noticed the problem in your bathroom mirror. In other words, consider how the American physique has changed over the years.

In the 19th century, few people in this country worried about their waistlines. It's not that our ancestors didn't care about their weight. The fact is, fat people were extremely rare, typically found among the upper class. After all, only the wealthy could afford to overindulge in rich, decadent foods back then. In 1890, for example, a survey of more than 5,000 white males in their fifties found that just 3.4 percent were obese.

However, that once-lean population has gone the way of hoop dresses and top hats. Today, 32 percent of Americans are obese. What's more, according to the Centers for Disease Control and Prevention, an additional one-third of Americans are overweight, meaning they are not quite obese but still have an unhealthy amount of body fat. When you do the math, it adds up to an alarming problem: Two-thirds of Americans are either obese or overweight. However, unlike in the 19th century, weight problems afflict all segments of the population—rich and poor, young and old, every race and educational background. The nation's schoolyards may offer the most disturbing view of this epidemic: One in three children in the United States is overweight or obese.

Doctors and public health authorities are alarmed by the nation's growing girth for good reason. Carrying around excess weight increases the risk for deadly conditions such as heart disease, diabetes, and kidney disease. What's more, being fat in a culture that idolizes slender and beautiful celebrities can be psychologically crippling. But what's most worrisome, and most puzzling, is why obesity rates are rising so rapidly. On the eve of the American bicentennial—in 1975, when the nation had been in existence for nearly 200 years—the obesity rate in the United States reached 15 percent. Since then, in a period of just 30 years, the obesity rate more than *doubled*.

Why? What has caused America to become so flabby so fast?

Frustrated dieters often blame their genes. Perhaps you have tried to lose weight in the past, but you couldn't shed those extra pounds. Or maybe you managed to trim down, but the weight eventually returned. If so, in the back of your mind, you may have been tempted to blame your parents. After all, if you have your mother's eyes or your father's smile, doesn't it make sense that you got your chunky thighs or bulging belly from them, too?

In fact, scientists have isolated genes that may be linked to obesity. But we merely inherit a *tendency* for one body shape or another from our parents. Whether or not you become overweight and obese depends largely on the lifestyle choices you make—that is, what foods you eat and how much exercise you get. Further, when you consider the bigger picture, it's hard to imagine how genetics could possibly be blamed for the current rapid rise in obesity. After all, the human genetic code dates back millennia. Has some mutation in the human genome occurred across the US population during the past 3 or 4 decades that is causing widespread uncontrollable weight gain? That's highly unlikely. In fact, such a genetic alteration would have to be occurring in populations all over the world, because obesity rates are rising in countries across the globe.

Instead, something must have changed in our environment that is exploiting the human tendency to accumulate body fat. A couple of obvious candidates come to mind. For instance, you no longer need to be wealthy to eat a waist-expanding diet. Thanks to advances in farming, manufacturing, and shipping, delicious high-calorie foods are cheap and widely available. Meanwhile, Americans burn fewer calories each day than our ancestors did, due to the rise of laborsaving devices, from the lawn mower to the laptop computer.

But while there is no doubt that Americans eat too much and don't exercise enough, I believe that some other mechanism has contributed to the disturbing and unprecedented weight gain that has swept across the United States in recent years. Reams of data that have emerged from research labs over the past decade indict a specific food: a common form of sugar called fructose that most of us eat every day.

Americans consume 30 percent more fructose today than in 1970. Our rising consumption of this sugar began at roughly the same time that obesity rates in the United States were climbing sharply. In the pages that follow, I will explain why I believe these corresponding trends are intimately linked—why feeding on so much fructose is fueling a public health catastrophe in the United States, and how you can lose weight and safeguard your overall health by limiting your exposure to this dangerous sweetener.

The Fructose Connection

Fructose has always been part of the human diet, since the first hungry forager plucked an apple from a tree or berries from a bush. That's because fructose, as the name suggests, is the main form of sugar found in fruit. Honey is another abundant natural source. What's more, half of every crystal of refined sugar consists of fructose, too.

If you have read much about fructose lately, that's probably because it is the critical component in a controversial sweetener called high-fructose corn syrup (HFCS), which is used in a wide variety of processed foods and beverages. Most brands of soda and many kinds of candy contain HFCS. If you were to start reading product labels, you'd find that HFCS is also in many foods that might surprise you, such as pasta sauce, yogurt, soups, ketchup and other condiments, and sandwich bread. In 1970, the average American consumed less than ½ pound of HFCS per year. By 2000, per capita consumption of the corn-based sweetener had risen to more than 42 pounds per year.

Critics call HFCS "Frankensyrup" and other damning names, blaming it for the current outbreak of obesity, especially among children in the United States. In later chapters, I'll examine HFCS more closely and sort out some of the claims its defenders and detractors have made. For now, though, here's the important point: There is mounting scientific evidence that consuming too much fructose, no matter where it comes from, can make you fat and increase your risk for high blood pressure, heart disease, diabetes, and kidney disease.

Fructose and Your Waistline

In the past generation, scientists from all over the world have begun to closely examine fructose and its effects on human health. My colleagues and I are actively involved in this research. We have made a number of discoveries about changes that occur in the body from consuming fructose and certain other foods and how they can cause weight gain and health problems. Our work, along with investigations conducted by other scientists, strongly suggests that America's fondness for fructose-rich foods is fueling the obesity epidemic. I will discuss these findings in greater detail throughout this book, but here is a snapshot of what we have learned so far.

Eating a high-fructose diet causes rapid weight gain. Eating too much of any form of sugar will make you fat. However, recent studies—performed in my laboratory, as well as by other scientists—have found that animals gain weight very quickly and develop other unhealthy symptoms when they eat too much fructose. Yet the same thing does *not* occur when animals are fed equal amounts of other sugars. In fact, eating fructose causes far more accumulation of abdominal fat—the most dangerous kind—than other forms of sugar, *even if the same number of calories is consumed.*

High-fructose foods do not satisfy your appetite. When you eat most types of sugar, your body responds by producing appetite hormones, which signal your brain that your body has consumed enough food to meet its energy needs. As this occurs, feelings of hunger subside. But unlike other sugars, fructose escapes the attention of appetite hormones. Because of this phenomenon, your brain never gets the message that your body has consumed a load of calories. As a result, the appetite center in your brain remains unsatisfied, so you continue eating. In one study, subjects felt hungrier after drinking beverages sweetened with fructose than they did after drinking beverages that contained another simple sugar, glucose. This may mean that fructose tricks you into eating more calories than your body needs. The result? You gain weight.

High-fructose foods may interfere with the signaling system that controls your appetite for *all* foods. We have discovered another way in which a high-fructose diet encourages overeating. Chronic consumption of sugary foods seems to promote biochemical changes that prevent the brain from receiving messages from appetite hormones—even when you are not consuming fructose. We have shown that this phenomenon leads to substantial weight gain in animals, and some studies suggest that it occurs in humans who consume too much fructose, too.

Fructose may sabotage weight-loss efforts. Your body does not metabolize fructose in the same way that it processes other sugars. When fructose enters a cell, enzymes break it down. Unfortunately, the actions of these enzymes raise blood pressure, increase blood levels of artery-clogging fat, and eventually cause obesity. As if that weren't bad enough, eating fructose actually increases your body's production of the very enzymes that cause all of these problems. Over time, your body may produce such a high concentration of these enzymes that eating foods that contain even a small amount of fructose will set in motion all of the powerful biological changes that we believe cause obesity, cardiovascular disease, diabetes, and other related conditions. This phenomenon may help explain why obese people struggle to lose weight and keep it off: Their bodies become ultraresponsive to fructose.

People who consume a lot of soft drinks and fruit juice—two major sources of fructose—tend to be overweight. Several large population studies have shown that people who drink beverages sweetened with fructose are more likely to be overweight than people who avoid soft drinks and juice. The "Supersize Me!" phenomenon is partly to blame. HFCS is cheaper than refined sugar, so fast-food restaurants and the beverage industry have been able to sell extra-large servings of soda and other fructose-rich beverages at low prices, which has led people to consume more calories. Soft drinks appear to pose another problem for anyone trying to control their weight and stay healthy. Consuming fructose rapidly—the way you might when gulping down a cola or bottle of fruit juice—causes levels of this sugar to soar in the blood. Studies suggest that could lead to greater weight gain.

Beyond Obesity

As every doctor learns in medical school, obesity raises the risk for many common conditions, including heart disease, high blood pressure, diabetes, and kidney disease, among others. As I just explained, strong evidence suggests that consuming too much fructose will make you gain an unhealthy amount of weight. Recent research has revealed that exposing the body to too much fructose makes you sick in other ways, independent of its effect on weight. In fact, I believe that consuming excessive amounts of fructose not only is making the United States one of the fattest nations in the world, but it also is hastening the rise of several of the leading killers in this country.

Indeed, even if you are currently eating a low-calorie diet and you are at a stable weight—or even if you are currently *losing* weight—you may still be creating health problems if your diet contains too much fructose. Actually, you could end up developing many of the complications associated with obesity, *even though you are not obese*. With this in mind, it's worth noting that rates of several other serious conditions, in addition to obesity, have soared at the same time that consumption of fructose has risen.

High blood pressure. Over the past 30 years, the number of Americans with high blood pressure has climbed by 20 percent. About 73 million people in this country have high blood pressure, also called hypertension, making it the most common disease in the United States. While hypertension often has no symptoms, it can have serious consequences, because it raises the risk for stroke, heart failure, and kidney disease.

Type 2 diabetes. The incidence of diabetes in the United States has increased by about 35 percent since 1994. A rare disease in this country as recently as the late 19th century, diabetes now affects more than 20 million Americans. New cases of type 2 diabetes account for almost all of this dramatic rise. This condition used to be called adult-onset diabetes, but its name was changed to reflect the unfortunate new reality: Like obesity and hypertension, type 2 diabetes has become commonplace among children and adolescents.

Kidney disease. During the past quarter-century, the incidence of end-stage renal disease, or kidney failure, has nearly quadrupled. Meanwhile, about 20 million Americans have mild to moderate degrees of kidney disease. Unfortunately, while treatment can slow its progression, there is little we can do to stop it completely.

Liver disease. In the past, a condition known as fatty liver occurred primarily in poorly nourished alcoholics. Now we know that too much nourishment—that is, overeating, which results in obesity—can cause a condition called nonalcoholic fatty liver disease (NAFLD). Once exceedingly rare, NAFLD now affects about 20 percent of Americans, including 6.5 million children. This disease can lead to complete liver failure and has become one of the most common reasons for liver transplantation. Recent studies by our group strongly suggest that consuming too much fructose may cause this condition.

Metabolic syndrome. Perhaps the best way to sum up the troubling state of overall health among Americans is to consider the rising number of adults in this country who have metabolic syndrome. Physicians use this term (which replaced *syndrome X*) to describe a cluster of conditions that includes obesity, high blood pressure, elevated blood fats, and insulin resistance. Having metabolic syndrome increases the risk for heart disease, strokes, diabetes, kidney disease, and other leading causes of death. During the 1990s, the portion of the American population with metabolic syndrome rose by a stunning 25 percent, to 55 million.

How do we know that consuming too much fructose is driving up rates of these various conditions? You could argue that these diseases are becoming more common simply because Americans are living longer. Thanks to the introduction of better public hygiene, immunizations, antibiotics, and other improvements to our health-care system over the past century, more people are living to ripe old ages. As the median age continues to rise in the United States—the oldest baby boomers turned 60 in 2006—a growing number of people are middle-aged or older, which is when many of us gain weight and develop features of metabolic syndrome.

That said, the current epidemic of obesity and metabolic syndrome in the United States and much of the world can't be blamed entirely on aging. If that were true, only older people would be getting fatter and sicker. To see that this is not the case, visit an elementary school or sit in the waiting room of a pediatric clinic. Obesity, hypertension, diabetes, and kidney disease are becoming more common among people of all ages, including our children. In other words, we're getting fatter and sicker not because we're living longer but because of how we live.

High-Fructose Fallout

If fructose were on trial, then so far all we'd have is circumstantial evidence against it. We know that rates of obesity and metabolic syndrome have multiplied in this country at the same time that Americans have been on a fructose binge. But that's not enough to prove that this sugar is the guilty party. To demonstrate that consuming too much fructose is contributing to ill health, we need to know *how* it causes metabolic problems in the first place. Fortunately, we're learning more every day about fructose's dark side. For example, studies show the following:

A high-fructose diet causes high blood pressure. Overloading the body with fructose raises blood pressure. As we will discuss in later chapters, this seems to occur because fructose increases blood levels of a compound called uric acid. Other forms of sugar do not raise uric acid, so they do not appear to have any effect on blood pressure.

A high-fructose diet raises levels of unhealthy blood fats. Fructose causes liver cells to produce triglycerides, a type of blood fat. Fructose also lowers HDL cholesterol, which is the "good" kind of cholesterol that guards against heart disease. Other forms of sugar do not have this effect on the liver. By raising triglycerides and lowering HDL cholesterol, a high-fructose diet may lead to blockages in the arteries that promote heart disease. Eating a high-fructose diet may also increase deposits of triglycerides within liver cells, causing swelling and damage. Over time, this damage could lead to fatty liver disease and eventually cirrhosis.

A high-fructose diet causes insulin resistance. Eating fructose for extended periods can make cells less responsive to insulin. People who develop the condition known as insulin resistance are at increased risk for type 2 diabetes and high blood pressure.

A high-fructose diet causes kidney disease. We have evidence from animal studies indicating that fructose-rich diets cause kidney damage and worsen existing kidney disease. Other forms of sugar do not have this effect on kidneys. This discovery is particularly frightening given that physicians often advise patients with kidney disease to eat low-protein, high-carbohydrate diets, which could lead to increased fructose consumption.

The results of research on fructose have been remarkably consistent. While most of these investigations have involved laboratory animals, a growing body of research is demonstrating many of the same effects in humans, too. Meanwhile, millions of people are presently engaging in a massive, uncontrolled trial of fructose and its impact on the human body.

Humans have been consuming fructose for millennia, but it didn't come to play a major role in our diets until about a century ago. Since then, fructose consumption has risen sixfold in the United States. In the next chapter, I will examine how our diets became dominated by food and drink sweetened with the two major sources of fructose: sugar and HFCS.

CHAPTER 2

RAISING CANE

The Fructose Story

One day, about 10,000 years ago, a native walked along a riverbank in New Guinea, searching for something to eat. He came upon a tall, grassy plant with slender green leaves. Curious, the native broke off a piece of the fibrous stalk and chewed it. His mouth filled with a pleasing, nectar-like sensation. Brimming with excitement, he dashed home to tell his family and friends about this remarkable plant.

Granted, it's not as though CNN was on hand to record this historic event, so we can only speculate how the plant we now call sugarcane might have been discovered. Yet this momentous occasion changed the course of history. The craving for sugar would help shape the world economy, while bringing out the best and worst in humanity—inspiring chefs to create culinary wonders yet forcing entire populations into slavery in order to harvest this coveted food. Perhaps most important, the discovery of sugarcane ensured that humans would one day consume large quantities of a substance that our bodies are designed to process in small doses: fructose.

Each year, the typical American consumes about 60 pounds of fructose. For perspective, consider that every citizen of this nation of Big Mac and Whopper lovers eats about 62 pounds of beef and 31 pounds of cheese annually. We wash down burgers and other fast-food treats with fructose-rich soda, of course. As you'll see, this sweetener has become omnipresent in the American diet. Many critics are fond of saying that fructose is in *everything* these days. That's an exaggeration, but even health-conscious people who watch what they eat may be consuming large amounts of fructose each day without realizing it.

Sweet Talk

Fructose, as you by now know, is a type of sugar. For most people, the word *sugar* calls to mind the familiar white crystals that we stir into coffee or tea. But sugar takes many forms, and it's important to understand how they are alike and how they differ.

Sugar is a carbohydrate, which is one of the three major types of nutrients in the human diet. (The other two are fat and protein.) The simplest forms of sugar, which can't be broken down into smaller sugars, are known as monosaccharides. Fructose is a monosaccharide, as is glucose, another form of sugar you have probably heard of. Most other sugars are disaccharides, which are combinations of monosaccharides. For instance, table sugar, also known as sucrose, is a combination of one fructose molecule and one glucose molecule.

There are other sugars, such as lactose (a combination

of glucose and galactose), which is found in milk. But this book will focus primarily on fructose, glucose, and sucrose. Throughout these pages, when I use the term *sugar*, I will be referring broadly to all sweeteners in foods, including naturally occurring sugars and manufactured additives, such as high-fructose corn syrup (HFCS). When I'm discussing sucrose, I'll usually use the terms *table sugar* or *refined sugar*. (In case you were wondering, confectioners' sugar and brown sugar—which are common ingredients in baking—are simply different forms of sucrose.)

All sugars share a few things in common. For starters, they provide fuel for your body—about 4 calories per gram, which is the same amount as protein and half as much as fats. All sugars share another obvious trait: They taste sweet. However, they vary greatly in *how* sweet they taste. Fructose is the sweetest sugar of all. Glucose is approximately 50 to 60 percent as sweet as fructose, while sucrose falls somewhere between the two—about 70 to 85 percent as sweet as fructose.

As you learned in the introduction, fructose is the main sugar in fruit. (It is sometimes called fruit sugar or levulose.) Vegetables contain smaller amounts of fructose. Honey, meanwhile, is one of the most concentrated natural sources of the sugar, containing about 70 percent fructose.

Today, the majority of fructose in most diets comes from added sweeteners. One source is obvious, because fructose molecules make up half of every crystal of table sugar. What's more, many processed foods and beverages are sweetened with HFCS. Despite its somewhat misleading name, most HFCS used in commercial food and beverage manufacturing does not have an unusually high amount of fructose. In fact, HFCS has roughly the same proportion of fructose and glucose as table sugar.

Sweetness: A Hardwired Preference

Fruit and vegetables are plant foods that provide plenty of health benefits. But parents often must plead with children to eat their vegetables, and many people carry that distaste into adulthood. (President George H. W. Bush, you may recall, detested broccoli so much that he had it removed from the White House menu during his term in office.) On the other hand, few people need to be coaxed into eating a crisp apple, juicy orange, or ripe banana. Why do we love fruit so much? Probably due to its abundance of sweet-tasting fructose.

Indeed, humans appear to be hardwired to seek out and devour sweet foods, as I will discuss in Chapter 6. For instance, studies show that newborns prefer sugary water to plain unflavored water. This natural yearning for sweet foods exists across our extended family, so to speak; studies of modern apes have shown that our fellow primates crave fruit, too.

No one can say for sure why humans developed a love for sweet foods. This inborn taste preference may have been an important survival mechanism for our early ancestors. After all, fruit and other natural sources of fructose are rich in life-sustaining nutrients. What's more, fructose-rich foods promote weight gain because they tend to be high in calories and—as I'll explain later—they do a poor job of satisfying appetite, so they encourage overeating.

How would a high-calorie food that makes you want to keep eating improve survival? Putting on a few extra pounds whenever possible may have made sense for early humans trying to survive from meal to meal. If the hunt failed or famine struck, carrying a little extra fat would have provided a sustaining source of energy until more food became available. Just as bears seek out and gorge on fructose-rich honey before they hibernate, our ancestors may have filled up on ripening fruit to gain weight as insurance against starvation before the long, barren winter months.

Experimental studies also suggest that eating fructose-rich foods may raise blood pressure, which could have conferred another unexpected benefit to early humans. How could this be? After all, high blood pressure is one of the most common, and troublesome, medical conditions in the United States today. But our ancestors may have struggled at times with the opposite problem—excessively low blood pressure, known as hypotension.

As you may know, eating too much sodium from salty foods causes high blood pressure in some people. But the body requires a minimal amount of sodium to maintain normal blood pressure. Anthropological studies suggest that the diets of early humans contained little sodium. Because very low blood pressure is unhealthy, humans who had access to foods that offset the relative lack of sodium had an advantage in survival. Fructose-rich foods offered just such an advantage, because they create changes in the body that raise blood pressure. What was once a biological edge, though, is now a major health threat.

Our cave-dwelling ancestors may have craved sweet foods all the more intensely simply because they were so hard to come by. Although fructose-rich fruit has probably been part of the human diet since the dawn of time, it was not cultivated until about 6,000 years ago (dates and figs may have been the earliest fruit crops). Our oldest ancestors were probably limited to whatever fruit they could gather from trees and bushes near their settlements. Because they had no way to preserve or store fruit for long periods, these sweet foods were a relatively infrequent treat, not part of the daily diet.

Cave drawings in Spain that date back to about 8000 BC appear to show people raiding beehives for honey. But honey was difficult (to say nothing of dangerous) to obtain, and it would be centuries before mass-production techniques made it a common food. Given how special fruit and honey must have seemed to our forebears, it's no wonder Greek mythology depicts these treasures as foods of the gods.

We can't be sure how much fructose our primitive ancestors ate every day, but it was probably very little— perhaps just 15 to 20 grams at the most, or about the amount in one or two pieces of fruit. Today, the typical American consumes approximately 70 to 80 grams of fructose per day, though people who eat a lot of processed and fast foods may consume far more. In fact, up to $\frac{1}{5}$ of the US population gets 15 to 20 percent, if not more, of its total calories in the form of fructose.

Thanks to modern refrigeration, food processing, and worldwide shipping, fruit and honey are no longer rare pleasures. They are available in any grocery store, year-round. Further, only a fraction of our fructose intake comes from these natural sources. The reason Americans and people all over the world consume so much more fructose today than our early ancestors did—far more than Americans consumed just a century ago, in fact—is that our diets often include huge doses of refined sugar, HFCS, and other added sweeteners.

Honey Without Bees

Humans are an industrious and determined species. From the moment one of our distant ancestors discovered a plant with stalks that yielded an intensely sweet flavor, it was only a matter of time before someone figured out how to extract the source of that pleasant sensation. Thousands of years later, we're beginning to understand the price of our success.

As I mentioned earlier, common table sugar, or sucrose, is a carbohydrate made up of two simple sugars, fructose and glucose. All plants produce sucrose, but a few contain very large quantities. Natives in the land now called New Guinea, the massive island north of Australia, discovered a tropical grass that came to be known as sugarcane, perhaps around 8000 BC. The sweet-tasting stalks were eventually carried to other lands, including India, where juices pressed from sugarcane were first boiled to produce crystals. Darius the Great discovered sugarcane in India while extending the reach of the Persian Empire, calling it "the reed that gives honey without bees." (This quote has also been attributed to a general in the army of Alexander the Great, who found sugarcane during his campaign in India.)

The Arabs discovered sugar when they invaded Persia in the 7th century. Soon the sweet crystals spread throughout much of the land we now call the Middle East, as well as Spain and Crete. Europeans brought home tales of an exotic new spice during the Crusades, and the first recorded reference to sugar in England dates back to 1099. The sugar trade flourished, though the sweet crystals were strictly a luxury item that only the wealthy could afford. In fact, most of the sugar produced during this era was used not in cooking, but as medicine. One historical reference from 1319 notes that a pound of sugar sold in London for the equivalent of about $50 in modern US currency.

By the late 1400s, Spain and Portugal began growing sugarcane. The new crop produced so much wealth that Portugal's King Emmanuel I (1469–1521), who was known as the Fortunate, sent life-size sugar effigies of the cardinals and the pope to the Vatican as gifts.

Christopher Columbus expanded worldwide sugar production when he brought sugarcane to the island of Hispaniola, which is occupied now by Haiti and the Dominican Republic, on his second voyage in 1493. Sugar plantations sprang up throughout the Caribbean islands, the Guiana coasts, and Brazil, and eventually in the southern United States.

In 1505, one of most tragic chapters in the sugar story began as the first ship of African slaves departed for America to work on the plantations. The next $3\frac{1}{2}$ centuries witnessed the flourishing of the infamous Triangle Trade. Ships sailed from European ports to Africa loaded with goods such as brass, copper, lead, salt, and gunpowder. These commodities were used to purchase slaves, who were then shipped across the famed Middle Passage to sugar plantations in the Caribbean and the southern United States. Historians estimate that between 10 million and 20 million Africans were brought to America during this period. To complete the triangle, ships would return to Europe filled with cargo from the New World, including sugar and molasses, as well as rum, hemp, and tobacco.

By capturing the Spanish settlement of Kingston, Jamaica, and increasing domestic production, England eventually became Europe's main importer and manufacturer of sugar. But the English exported very little sugar to their neighbors. As a result, sugar became more widely available in England and commonly used to sweeten chocolates, teas, and cakes. At the dawn of the 18th century, per capita consumption of sugar in England was 4 pounds per year; that figure rose to 18 pounds by 1800.

Although the sweets-loving English hoarded sugar, other European countries soon had their own regular supply of the coveted sweetener. In 1747, a German scientist discovered that sucrose could be derived from beets, too. Soon farms growing "sugar beets" sprouted up in Germany and France. The treasure sometimes called white gold was becoming available to the masses, though it was no less precious.

Liquid Sugar: High-Fructose Corn Syrup

The colonists who left England for new lives across the Atlantic carried with them a love of sweet foods. The earliest versions of the confections we know as candy bars became available in the early 19th century. These treats were too expensive for most Americans until a drop in the price of sugar after World War I lowered their cost to just a nickel.

Sweetened soft drinks were popular in the United States by the 1830s, and the first glass of a beverage that came to be called Coca-Cola was poured in an Atlanta pharmacy in 1886. Many more would follow, of course. Today, Americans drink more than 10 billion cases of carbonated beverages per year.

An event that occurred 20 years earlier, in 1866, may have had an equally profound impact on the American diet and your health. Food scientists at a manufacturing plant in Buffalo, New York, used techniques that had been pioneered a few decades earlier to turn corn into sugar. Specifically, they converted cornstarch into sweet-tasting corn syrup.

In a sense, this impressive act of alchemy is rather simple. The starchy portion of foods such as corn, potatoes, and wheat is made up of long chains of glucose molecules. The reason starch does not taste sweet is that these chains are too large to fit into the sweetness receptors on the tongue. By breaking these chains, however, we can change the way starch tastes. As a child, you may have done the schoolroom experiment that demonstrates this phenomenon. Place a plain cracker in your mouth, but don't chew it. At first, the cracker tastes bland. Within a moment or two, though, saliva breaks down the glucose chains, and suddenly the cracker tastes sweet.

Processing cornstarch with acids and enzymes has a similar effect, breaking up chains of glucose molecules to produce a sweet syrup. If you like to bake, you may have a bottle of corn syrup in your cupboard. Food manufacturers began using corn syrup in a wide variety of products in the 1920s. But simple corn syrup has several drawbacks that limit its usefulness. The biggest problem: Corn syrup contains no fructose, which means that it is far less sweet than table sugar. So while corn syrup is a useful additive in recipes, it cannot replace refined sugar in food.

Scientists overcame this problem in the 1960s when they discovered that treating corn syrup with an enzyme called glucose isomerase converts some of its glucose to fructose. The new technique was expensive, so initially it was not practical for food processing. That all changed in 1971, when two Japanese scientists found a way to reuse the critical enzymes by attaching them to a column through which corn syrup was poured. This innovation allowed refiners to convert corn to a blend of glucose and fructose at a lower cost.

Within a few years, the food industry began replacing some of the sugar it used with the new product, HFCS. Though scientists can alter the fructose content of HFCS to vary its sweetness, the most common versions of this food additive in manufacturing taste about as sweet as refined sugar.

HFCS has other qualities that make it appealing to food and beverage manufacturers. For instance, it dissolves more readily in other liquids than refined sugar or plain corn syrup does. It doesn't spoil easily, so it prolongs the shelf life of foods. If you ever bit into a stale chocolate bar as a child, you may remember seeing that crystals had formed inside. That's less likely to happen today, because most chocolate bars are sweetened with HFCS. The makers of ice cream and other frozen desserts appreciate this quality, too, because sugar crystallization often occurs at low temperatures, resulting in freezer burn. Product designers say that HFCS makes foods softer and chewier than sugar does.

HFCS has other attributes that make it useful to the makers of products we don't normally think of as sweet. For example, much of the bread you'll find in your local supermarket is baked with HFCS, which gives its crust an appealing brown burnish. Start reading the ingredients lists on product labels, and you will discover that HFCS appears in a remarkable array of foods. (See "The Ubiquitous Sweetener.")

Food scientists may appreciate the unique qualities of

HFCS, but it became food processors' sweetener of choice because company accountants liked its low price. HFCS costs less than refined sugar for several reasons. For starters, the US government subsidizes corn growers, who in turn plant lots of the crop—more than 80 million acres, which would nearly fill the state of New Mexico. Corn on the cob and creamed corn may be popular dishes, but 80 million acres produces far more ears than farmers could ever sell as food. The glut leads to low prices and plenty of bushels available for corn refiners to turn into HFCS, among myriad other products (such as animal feed, corn oil, and ethanol, to name just a few). About 5 percent of the corn grown in the United States goes toward the production of HFCS.

By the late 1970s, Americans were consuming about 10 pounds of HFCS per person each year. Yet food processors still used six times more refined sugar than HFCS. Although HFCS was inexpensive to produce, sugar was a relatively cheap commodity at the time, too. A major turning point in the HFCS story occurred in 1982, when Congress enacted strict limits on the amount of sugar that could be imported into the United States, driving up its price. The law was ostensibly intended to protect domestic sugar producers from foreign competition—but corn refiners benefited from the quotas, too, which ensure that HFCS will always be cheaper than imported sugar.

In November 1984, 2 years after the US Congress set limits on sugar imports, the makers of Coca-Cola and Pepsi announced on the same day that they planned to replace refined sugar with HFCS in their regular and caffeine-free soft drinks. Today, most soft drinks sold in the United States are sweetened with HFCS.

HFCS and the Supersizing of America

If you read newspapers, watch television, or browse the Internet, you probably already know that HFCS is controversial. Critics have blamed it for the obesity epidemic. Type "high-fructose corn syrup" into an Internet search engine, and you will find plenty of Web sites that demonize HFCS. Many people insist that their health improved dramatically when they stopped consuming HFCS.

That's all nonsense, insist representatives for the corn-refining industry, who say that condemning HFCS is unfair. After all, they point out, the most commonly used forms of this liquid sweetener have virtually the same chemical structure as table sugar. As I explained earlier, sucrose, or table sugar, consists of equal parts fructose and glucose. One of the most widely used forms of HFCS—the sweetener in most carbonated soft drinks—is 55 percent fructose and 45 percent glucose. So this sweetener, known as HFCS-55, contains slightly more fructose than table sugar does, but not much. Meanwhile, manufacturers often use a product called HFCS-42 to sweeten many noncarbonated fruit drinks and other foods. As you might guess, it has only 42 percent fructose, or 8 percentage points *less* than table sugar.

Though some HFCS has more fructose than table sugar and some has less, surveys suggest that it all balances out in the end. That is, if you combine all of the HFCS-55 and HFCS-42 Americans consume, roughly half of it consists of fructose. In other words, HFCS is really no different from table sugar, the corn refiners claim. So why blame it for the fattening of America?

It's absolutely true that the table sugar you sprinkle in

THE UBIQUITOUS SWEETENER

Food processors may use high-fructose corn syrup (HFCS) in the following products, according to the Corn Refiners Association.

Asian-style sauces

Baby foods

Bacon

Beer

Biscuits

Bologna

Brandy

Breads and rolls

Breakfast cereals

Breakfast meats

Cake and dessert mixes

Cakes

Candy

Canned fruits and fruit fillings

Canned vegetables

Caramel coloring

Carbonated beverages (nondiet)

Cat and dog foods

Cheese spreads

Chewing gum

Chicken products

Cocoa

Coffee creamer

Cookies

Cordials

Crackers

Dessert toppings

Diet foods

Doughnuts

Dried meats

Egg products

Fish products

Flavorings

Frosting, icing, glazes

Frozen dinners

Frozen puddings and custards

Fruit butters

Fruit drinks and juices

Fruit sweeteners

Gelatin mixes

Gravies

Ham

Hot dogs

Ice cream or milk

Instant breakfast foods

Instant tea

Jams

Jellies

Ketchup

Liqueurs

Low-calorie sweeteners

Marmalade

Mayonnaise

Mincemeat

Mustard

Pancake, waffle mixes

Peanut butter

Pickles

Pies

Potato chips

Powdered mixes

Powdered sugar

Preserves

Pretzels

Quickbread mixes

Relishes

Salad dressings

Sauce mixes

Sausage

Seasoning mixes

Sherbets, water ices

Soups, canned or dried

Tomato sauces

Vinegar

Wine

Worcestershire sauce

Yeast

Source: Nutritive Sweeteners from Corn, *2006, Corn Refiners Association*

HFCS AND REFINED SUGAR: ARE THEY REALLY THE SAME?

Food chemists may say that HFCS and table sugar are practically identical, but some food lovers disagree. "My own case against high-fructose corn syrup is that what little flavor it has is strangely violent," observed *Atlantic Monthly* food writer Corby Kummer, in an article about commercially brewed iced tea. "Drinks sweetened with corn syrup taste like only their usual artificial flavorings, and the effect is a clobbering sweetness, as if someone had come up behind you, held your nose, and poured syrup down your throat."

---

your coffee or add to your cookie batter has a chemical structure nearly identical to that of HFCS: Both are roughly equal parts fructose and glucose. The real problem with HFCS may not be its chemistry (though we'll examine that issue later on). The greater concern may be one of economics. HFCS's low price appears to have allowed the food and beverage industry to market sweet-tasting products more aggressively. As a result, Americans consume greater amounts of fructose, which has led to higher rates of obesity and all sorts of other serious metabolic problems.

Let's back up for a moment. Defenders of HFCS claim that it has simply replaced an equal amount of table sugar in food processing. Statistics from the USDA tell another story. As the accompanying chart shows, the total amount of sugar consumed in this country, per person, has increased significantly since the introduction of HFCS.

PER CAPITA CONSUMPTION OF REFINED SUGAR AND HFCS		
	1970	2004
Refined sugar	72.5 lb	44 lb
HFCS	0.4 lb	42.3 lb
Refined sugar and HFCS combined	72.9 lb	86.3 lb

In 1970, the typical American consumed slightly less than 73 pounds of refined sugar and HFCS combined. By 2004, according to USDA data, that figure had jumped to more than 86 pounds per person. This means that intake of refined sugar and HFCS—and therefore fructose—rose by more than 18 percent in a quarter-century.

There is good reason to believe that this estimate is too low by nearly half—that Americans actually increased their fructose intake even more than the government statistics suggest. The USDA calculates the amount of sugar each American consumes by using a formula based on a number of variables, including how much sugar is actually sold, how much may be wasted, and so on. A different picture of our sugar consumption emerges from diet surveys, in which researchers interview large numbers of people to find out what they eat every day.

Using data from diet surveys conducted by the federal government, researchers Barry Popkin, PhD, and George Bray, MD, determined that the typical American consumed about 158.5 calories of fructose from sweeteners per day in the late 1970s. That figure includes only the fructose in table sugar and in HFCS (excluding the more modest amounts in fruit, honey, and other foods). By the mid-1990s, according to Drs. Popkin and Bray, the daily intake of fructose per American had risen to 228 calories—a jump of 30 percent.

Where did all that extra fructose come from? Drs. Popkin and Bray lay much of the blame on HFCS, which appears to have helped promote the popularity of so-called supersize products, especially soft drinks. HFCS costs less than sugar, so when makers of soda and fruit juices started to use the sweetener, they could have passed their savings on to consumers in the form of lower prices. Instead, they dramatically increased the size of their offerings while raising prices only modestly. As author Greg Critser notes in his book *Fat Land*, switching to the cheaper HFCS was a critical move for Coca-Cola and PepsiCo that "saved both companies 20 percent in sweetener costs, allowing them to boost portion sizes and still make substantial profits."

A windfall for beverage makers, to be sure, but supersizing has been a mixed blessing for consumers—that is, you and your family. Although soda lovers can get more for their dollar, these oversize drinks entice people into consuming more calories and more fructose. If you're old enough, you may recall that back in the 1950s, a bottle of Coca-Cola contained just 6.5 ounces of the caramel-colored drink. That's puny compared with the 12-ounce bottles and cans that eventually replaced them. Now both are dwarfed by the hefty 20-ounce bottles that have become the standard single-serving size.

Even these bigger bottles seem like a drop in the bucket compared with the fountain drinks sold in fast-food restaurants, movie theaters, and convenience stores. The 7-Eleven chain took this trend to extremes with its Big Gulp fountain beverage, which is sold in 32-, 44-, 52-, and 64-ounce cups. (In 2005, the chain even introduced a Team Gulp drink, sold in a container that could hold 1 gallon—128 ounces—of soda and ice.) Many restaurants take the concept of supersizing a giant leap further by offering customers the chance to refill their huge cups as often as they wish for no additional charge.

Beverage industry officials have defended the supersizing of soft drinks by claiming that they are merely responding to the market: Consumers wanted bigger cups and bottles, so we made them. True or not, the bottom line is the same: Americans are consuming more soda and fruit juice today than a generation ago. Dr. Popkin and his colleagues at the University of North Carolina determined that today the typical American drinks 56 gallons of soft drinks per year. That's an increase of *70 percent* since 1977.

Much of the concern about the rising consumption of sweetened drinks in the United States has focused on young people. And with good reason: One study found that adolescent boys and girls, for example, get 14 to 16 percent of their calories from fructose. But there's a good chance you may be satisfying your daily thirst with more fructose-filled soda and fruit juice than ever, too.

When Dr. Popkin and researcher Kiyah J. Duffey analyzed government data, they discovered that American

A LOT TO SWALLOW

According to the USDA, fountain drinks—that is, soda poured from dispensers at fast-food restaurants and convenience stores—actually have less sugar than the same varieties sold in bottles and cans. But these mega products more than make up for this difference by virtue of their size.

Later in the book, I will explain why you should consume only 25 to 35 grams of fructose per day. Here, I list the fructose content of typical fountain drinks. As you can see, a single cup of cola can drain your fructose budget for a day—or much more.

FOUNTAIN DRINK SIZE (OZ)	FRUCTOSE CONTENT (G)
16	26.1
32	52.5
40	65.5
44	71.8
52	84.8

adults today are getting more of their daily calories from beverages than ever before. In fact, more than one in three adults consumes at least 25 percent of his or her calories in liquid form. In the 1970s, that was true of only about one person in seven.

Unfortunately, much of the increase in beverage consumption has come from soda and fruit drinks. Between 1977 and 2002, the typical American adult upped his or her daily intake of soda by 157 calories. That's like drinking an additional 12-ounce can of cola every day. If you don't like soda, perhaps you're drinking more fruit juice. While we associate fruit-flavored beverages with children, over the past generation, the typical American adult has added about 100 calories from juice drinks to his or her daily diet.

About two-thirds of the fructose Americans consume comes from carbonated beverages and fruit drinks. But as HFCS has become a stealth ingredient in so many foods, you may have increased your intake of fructose in recent years even if you don't like sweetened drinks.

The Real Price of Fructose

To sum up: Early humans ate very little fructose. Their main sources were the limited amounts of fruits and vegetables they were able to forage. As recently as a century ago, sugar and other sources of fructose played a minor role in most diets. Today, fructose is present, often in large quantities, in a stunning array of foods. Walk down virtually any aisle in a modern supermarket, and you will find products sweetened with fructose. (That includes the pharmacy aisle, as even some cough syrup contains HFCS, for example.) As a result, I estimate that we consume five to seven times more fructose today than our primitive ancestors did. Much of the huge increase in fructose consumption in the American diet has occurred in the past generation.

So? Why does it matter whether you consume a little fructose or a lot?

The species *Homo sapiens* has walked the earth for at least 130,000 years, possibly for as long as 195,000 years. Remarkably, our genetic makeup has not changed much in all that time. But our diets have changed, dramatically so. That's obvious enough—a caveman wouldn't know what to make of baked lasagna or a fried chicken dinner, of course. More to the point, the composition of basic nutrients that most people eat today is vastly different from what early humans consumed, or even what the typical American ate a century ago.

One of the most critical differences concerns our sugar intake. Simply put, the body you were born with was designed to run efficiently on small doses of fructose, not the massive load that many people consume each day. In the next chapter, I'll examine how the introduction of fructose-rich sugar into the human diet has affected our health.

CHAPTER 3

SWEET AND DANGEROUS

Fructose's Powerful Impact on Populations

When you add table sugar to a dish or beverage, it becomes sweet. Unfortunately, when you add table sugar and other sources of fructose to a population's daily diet, things turn sour in a hurry.

Consider the fate of the Maori, an indigenous tribe in New Zealand. Between AD 800 and AD 1300, the original Maori people migrated from other parts of Polynesia and settled on the two large islands that form this country in the southwestern Pacific Ocean. For centuries, the Maori were a lean, athletic population who ate diets consisting largely of fish, taro, sweet potato, and fern root. Then in the 19th century, European settlers began to arrive in New Zealand, and intermarriage between the Maori and the colonists became common. Many of the Maori adopted Western-style diets, which included large quantities of a food that was not previously an important part of their culinary heritage: sugar.

Within a short period, the Maori became some of the most obese people in the world. The prevalence of diabetes and hypertension, once virtually nonexistent in this population, soared. The problem has only worsened over time. Today, about one in four Maori adults has diabetes. What's more, the Maori, especially males, have some of the highest rates of cardiovascular disease in the world.

The situation is not quite so dire in the United States, but it's easy to look at the Maori experience as a microcosm of what has happened in this country and much of the world over the past century or so. As I explained in the previous chapter, the diets of our distant ancestors included only modest amounts of fructose. Since the 19th century, however, major sources of this monosaccharide—including table sugar, high-fructose corn syrup (HFCS), fruit, and honey—have become commonplace in the diets of Americans. Fructose consumption, in particular, has skyrocketed over the past 3 decades. And as our diets have become sweeter over time, we have gotten fatter and sicker.

Of course, our insatiable appetite for foods sweetened with table sugar, HFCS, and other sources of fructose is not the sole force that is driving the current epidemic of obesity, cardiovascular disease, diabetes, and other threats that lead to premature death. Americans also eat too many cheeseburgers, french fries, and other types of unhealthy foods. To be sure, most scientists, doctors, and policy makers in the United States have identified fat as the number-one dietary villain for the past half-century.

The case against sugar—and against fructose in particular—as a major health threat has been building for years. Much of the preliminary evidence comes from the field of epidemiology, the branch of medicine that examines the incidence and prevalence of disease in large populations, with an eye toward ferreting out potential causes. A number of epidemiological studies offer us a wealth of powerful clues, showing that people who consume large amounts of fructose tend to be overweight and have poor overall health.

It's important to recognize that epidemiological studies do not prove cause and effect. Rather, they show an association between two or more phenomena or trends. For example, epidemiological studies associated cigarette smoking with lung cancer. Similar research linked alcohol abuse to cirrhosis of the liver. And as I'll discuss later in this chapter, epidemiology made the early connection between high cholesterol and heart disease.

The epidemiological evidence linking a high-fructose diet to weight problems and other serious conditions is compelling—in fact, it's as strong as any of the other associations I mentioned. Researchers have shown repeatedly that the rise of sweet foods described in Chapter 2 occurred at the same time that Americans got fatter and new diseases emerged in the United States and throughout much of the world.

The Origins of an Epidemic

The news media has latched onto the idea that large numbers of Americans suddenly started gaining weight in the past few years. While that may be true, there is evidence to suggest that the origins of the obesity epidemic date back much further, to the 19th century. For example, a study of Civil War veterans in 1880 found that just 1.5 percent of the men were obese.

All things being equal, it's reasonable to suspect that a physical trait, such as body size, would remain stable and

THE PARALLEL RISE OF OBESITY
AND SUGAR INTAKE IN THE UNITED STATES

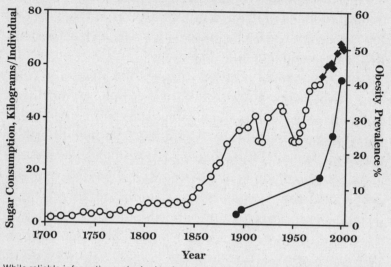

While reliable information on body size dates back only to the late 19th century, this chart shows that obesity rates have risen in parallel with sugar consumption for more than a century in the United States. The obesity rates (solid circles) are taken from weight measurements of men (average age 60). The sugar intake levels represent a composite of consumption levels in the United States (diamonds) and United Kingdom (open circles), which fell during both World Wars, yet eventually continued to rise and accelerated with the introduction of high-fructose corn syrup in the early 1970s.

Source: American Journal of Clinical Nutrition *86 (2007): 899–906. American Society for Nutrition.*

constant across a population over time. That has not been the case with the American physique. The portion of seriously overweight people in the United States doubled between 1880 and 1900, and obesity rates continued to climb steadily throughout the 20th century, to 14.5 percent in 1976. Since then, the portion of obese Americans has more than doubled, to the current 30 percent. In all, roughly two-thirds of our population is either obese or overweight.

As I explained in the previous chapter, sweet foods first became widely available in the United States in the mid-

1800s, with their popularity increasing as sugar prices dropped over time. Other than brief dips in consumption during World Wars I and II, our national intake of sugar rose year by year. With the introduction of HFCS in the early 1970s, the amount of table sugar the typical American consumed each year actually fell. Yet the total amount of fructose-rich sweeteners consumed rose steeply, as waistlines expanded and health worsened. (See the chart on page 39.)

Of course, much of that HFCS finds its way into soda, which accounts for 8 to 9 percent of the calories consumed by children and adults in this country. If you're like many people, you first became familiar with the phrase *high-fructose corn syrup* in 2004, when a headline-grabbing paper in the *American Journal of Clinical Nutrition* strongly suggested that an unquenchable thirst for soft drinks sweetened with HFCS was at least partly to blame for the epidemic of obesity in this country. The paper, written by George Bray, MD, Barry Popkin, PhD, and graduate student Samara Joy Nielsen, noted that consumption of HFCS increased *1,000-fold* in the United States between 1970 and 1990. "It is becoming increasingly clear that soft drink consumption may be an important contributor to the epidemic of obesity," Dr. Bray and his colleagues wrote. "If HFCS acts as an agent in the disease, then reducing exposure to this agent may help to reduce the epidemic."

To be fair, we don't know for certain whether HFCS is any more likely than refined sugar to make you gain weight or develop other health problems. The important point here is that a soft drink, whether sweetened with HFCS or refined sugar, is a delivery system for fructose. And studies tell us that people who drink a lot of sweetened beverages tend to gain weight.

For example, Harvard researchers tracked more than 50,000 women for several years, periodically asking them to fill out questionnaires describing their diets. They found that women who formerly drank few sugar-sweetened carbonated soft drinks but then began having one or more servings per day put on more than 17 pounds, on average, over an 8-year period. By comparison, most of the women who quit or cut back on soft drinks maintained a stable weight over the same period.

Another study, by David Ludwig, MD, and his colleagues at Children's Hospital in Boston, found that each sugar-sweetened beverage a child drinks is associated with a 60 percent increase in risk that he or she will become obese. While soda is obviously one of the most common

---

SHOULD YOU DRINK FRUIT JUICE?

It's portrayed in advertisements as wholesome and nutritious. But just how healthy is fruit juice?

First, the good news. Depending on which variety you choose, a glass of fruit juice may contain vitamin C, vitamin A, and other antioxidants, as well as potassium and other minerals. Some varieties have a small amount of protein. Others may be fortified with calcium.

That said, there are several good reasons to limit how much fruit juice you drink. For starters, the dominant sweetener in most juice is fructose. In fact, fruit juice usually has a much greater amount of this troublesome sugar than occurs naturally in whole fruit.

Only products that contain 100 percent fruit juice may bear the word "juice" on their labels. Fruit-flavored products that carry the words "drink," "beverage," "punch," or "cocktail" may contain very little real fruit. Instead, they are often sweetened with large amounts of HFCS or table sugar.

A number of studies have provided dramatic evidence indicating that drinking too much fruit juice can make children gain weight. The American Academy of Pediatrics advises parents to limit the amount of fruit juice they allow their children to consume to one serving (4 to 6 ounces) per day for children ages 1 to 6, two servings per day for children 7 to 18. As I will explain in Chapter 11, even that modest allowance may be too much.

sources of fructose, other beverages contain large concentrations of this sugar, too. For example, up to 60 to 65 percent of the calories in apple juice come from fructose.

Many parents continue to believe that it's better to give their children fruit juice instead of soda, even though compelling evidence suggests that consuming too much fructose from *any* source expands waistlines. A study published in the journal *Pediatrics* found that 32 percent of preschool children who drank more than 12 ounces of fruit juice per day were obese. Among children who drank less fruit juice, just 9 percent were dramatically overweight.

What makes this last study particularly interesting is that all the children involved consumed roughly the same number of calories in their overall diets, on average. So why did some become obese while others didn't? Fructose may have played a critical role. The children who consumed the most fruit juice were exposing their bodies to twice as much of this troublesome sugar as the others—and they were $3\frac{1}{2}$ times more likely to be obese. As I will explain soon, fructose has the uncanny ability to "trick" your body into gaining weight by fooling your metabolism.

More Than a Weight Problem

There is no doubt: People who consume diets rich in foods sweetened with table sugar, HFCS, and other sources of fructose tend to be overweight. But Americans did not merely become fatter as their sugar consumption rose. Our growing taste for sweet foods appears to have contributed to the rise of diseases that once were considered uncommon and exotic but that now represent the leading causes of death and disability in much of the world.

For example, though it seems hard to believe today, diabetes was an extremely rare disease just a century ago. There are two main forms of diabetes. Type 1 occurs when the pancreas is unable to produce insulin, the hormone that ushers glucose into cells. As a result, blood glucose levels rise and damage organs. In type 2, people can make insulin, but their cells resist its influence, which also results in high blood sugar. Left unchecked, elevated blood sugar can cause blindness, kidney disease, nerve damage, and a long list of other serious complications.

In 1893, there were fewer than two or three cases of diabetes per 100,000 people in the United States, according to a widely used medical text published that year. The author of the text, the famed physician William Osler, MD, noted that of 35,000 consecutive patients admitted to Johns Hopkins Hospital in Baltimore, just 10 had diabetes. Doctors of the day spent far more time treating patients sick with tuberculosis and other infectious diseases, which were the leading killers of the era.

That would all change in time, of course. Within 50 years, a million Americans had diabetes. Today, the figure has soared to more than 23 million. That works out to almost *8,000* cases per 100,000 people. Most major medical centers have entire clinics devoted to treating diabetes. The disease is a global problem, too—by one estimate, the worldwide incidence of diabetes will rise by 46 percent between 2000 and 2010.

Furthermore, in Dr. Osler's time, the form of diabetes now known as type 1 was by far the more common. Today, more than 90 percent of people diagnosed with the disease have type 2, the form that typically strikes people who are overweight or obese.

Large population studies show that people who consume a high-fructose diet often develop diabetes. For example, a

Harvard study of more than 90,000 female nurses found that women whose daily diets included one or more beverages sweetened with sugar or HFCS—both sources of fructose—had an 83 percent higher risk of developing type 2 diabetes.

The United States currently finds itself in the midst of a full-blown epidemic of type 2 diabetes. This insidious problem is not confined to our borders, however. Rising rates of diabetes have been detected in South America, India, and southeastern Asia, all parts of the world where sugar consumption has risen in recent years.

Along with diabetes, high blood pressure is another potentially devastating medical condition that made the transition from rare to rampant during the 20th century. Also called hypertension, high blood pressure is the leading cause of stroke and heart failure, and it raises the risk for heart attack, peripheral artery disease (hardening and narrowing of the arteries in the pelvis and legs), and kidney disease. Blood pressure is one of the first things your doctor checks during any physical exam, and for good reason: Hypertension is a silent killer.

The first cases of high blood pressure were described in England and Germany in the 1800s. Perhaps it's no coincidence that sugar intake rose in those two countries during that century. Interestingly, high blood pressure—like obesity—was a problem that primarily afflicted the wealthy, who could afford to buy sugar.

Nonetheless, hypertension remained a rare condition well into the 20th century. A study of more than 140,000 adults applying for life insurance in New York, conducted between 1907 and 1919, determined that only 5 to 6 percent had blood pressure of 140/90 mm Hg, which is the bench-

HEAD START ON HIGH BLOOD PRESSURE: CHILDREN AND HYPERTENSION

High blood pressure is becoming more common within one surprising population: children, who rarely were diagnosed with the condition in the past. Until recently, few people under age 40 developed essential hypertension, the most common form. When doctors detected elevated blood pressure in a young person, they assumed that the cause was a tumor or some form of vascular disease involving the kidneys.

We can no longer make that assumption. In a 2004 study published in the journal *Pediatrics*, researchers at the University of Texas measured the blood pressure of more than 5,000 children and teens between ages 10 and 19 at eight Houston public schools. Based on earlier estimates, they should have found that about 1 percent of these young people had elevated blood pressure. Instead, the figure was *four times* higher (4.5 percent).

Not surprisingly, hypertension was even more common among children who were severely overweight, of whom more than 1 in 10 had high blood pressure. Indeed, we suspect that obesity is to blame for about 50 percent of the incidence of hypertension we're seeing in adolescents today, which is rising along with our children's ever-growing intake of fructose from soda and sugary snacks.

mark for hypertension. The study was somewhat flawed, because it didn't include people who couldn't afford insurance or who were too ill to qualify. Still, it offers solid evidence that high blood pressure was at best a minor threat to public health in the United States prior to and during World War I.

Since that time, though, there has been a startling increase in blood pressure within the US population. In 1939, a study of more than 11,000 residents in the Chicago area found that 11 to 13 percent had high blood pressure. A 1975 study found that the prevalence of hypertension in the US population had jumped to 25 percent. Those rates have continued to climb. Today, 73 million Americans—roughly one in three adults—have high blood pressure.

The problem isn't unique to the United States, however. Hypertension became increasingly common in Europe, and particularly in England, France, and Germany, during the 20th century. Further, studies conducted as recently as 1940 show that certain populations in which high blood pressure once was virtually nonexistent—including Native Americans, Australian Aborigines, Alaskan Eskimos, Asians, and black Africans—have become much more likely to develop the condition as they've adopted Western-style diets.

Like obesity, hypertension is becoming a worldwide threat. According to one estimate, 29 percent of the world's population, or more than 1.5 billion people, will have high blood pressure by the year 2025.

Increases in diabetes and hypertension have also contributed to a striking rise in kidney disease. Although the body of historical data on the incidence of kidney disorders is smaller, we know that the incidence of end-stage renal disease—also known as kidney failure—has quadrupled in the United States over the past generation and that rates are climbing in other countries as well.

Heart Disease: The Surprising Role of Sugar

Of course, as America's appetite for sugar and other sources of fructose grew, cardiovascular disease rose from a medical rarity to the leading cause of death in the United States, now claiming more than 870,000 lives each year. This means that heart attacks and other cardiovascular disorders account for more than one in three deaths in this country today—which is all the more astonishing when you consider that they were infrequent just a century ago.

Coronary artery disease, the term for blockages in the

arteries that deliver blood to the heart, was not identified as a medical condition until 1914. Within a decade or so, family physicians were diagnosing the condition in a growing number of patients. By 1940, doctors agreed that the problem of heart disease had become important enough to spawn a new medical specialty, which became known as cardiology. Ten years later, there were 500 cardiologists in the United States. Since then, the general population of this country has doubled, yet the number of cardiologists has increased *60-fold*.

You may be wondering: What do sugar and other sources of fructose have to do with cardiovascular disease? After all, doesn't eating high-fat foods cause heart attacks? In fact, dietary fat first became linked to heart disease thanks to the very types of epidemiology studies I have discussed in this chapter (and which I'll describe further in

AFRICAN AMERICANS AND SUGAR

African Americans are more likely to be overweight and develop heart disease, high blood pressure, diabetes, and kidney disease than any other group in the United States. Many theories have been offered to explain these disparities.

The legacy of slavery may hold some answers. For example, some observers have noted that many of the 30 percent of African slaves who died on ships bound for America perished from conditions caused by dehydration. This suggests that Africans who were genetically predisposed to retain sodium, which prevents dehydration, were more likely to survive the voyage. Unfortunately, sodium retention also predisposes a person to developing high blood pressure.

It's also worth noting that many Africans brought to the United States as slaves worked on sugar plantations and in sugar houses. Molasses, the thick, fructose-rich by-product of sugar processing, became a staple of the early African American diet. Studies show that African Americans today consume more sugar than other groups. Perhaps not surprisingly, they also are more likely to be obese and to develop hypertension, type 2 diabetes, and kidney disease than Caucasian Americans.

Chapter 8). Because of these population studies, many cardiologists consider fat to be nutrition enemy number one. Meanwhile, most heart doctors pay far less attention to sugar. Tellingly, the American Heart Association's 2006 diet and lifestyle recommendations mention fat 127 times, compared with only 22 references to sugar.

Yet powerful scientific evidence from population, laboratory, and clinical research suggests that a diet high in sugar is bad for the heart—as bad as, or worse than, a diet high in fat. Much of the credit for calling attention to the role of sugar in heart disease goes to a British scientist and physician named John Yudkin, MD, who was a professor of nutrition and dietetics at the University of London. Dr. Yudkin did not dispute the epidemiological studies indicating that people who eat high-fat diets often develop heart disease. But he did show that people who eat a lot of fat also tend to consume large amounts of sugar. In fact, his data revealed that people who were diagnosed with cardiovascular disease ate more than twice as much sugar, on average, as people who were free of heart problems. Dr. Yudkin believed that sugar—which he called "pure, white, and deadly"—was probably a greater threat than fat.

Dr. Yudkin, who died in 1995, published several books, including *Sweet and Dangerous,* in which he linked sugar to many diseases and suggested banning the sweetener. He recommended a pre-Atkins version of the low-carb diet, though in the end, he was unable to convince the world that sugar was a greater threat to the heart than fat. The latter simply made more sense. After all, fat is a major component in atherosclerotic plaque, the blockages that clog arteries and cause heart attacks and strokes.

In his published work, Dr. Yudkin speculated that most

doctors and scientists failed to embrace his theories in part because he blamed sugar for so many different health woes, including heart disease, obesity, dental cavities, upset stomach, and skin rashes. Ultimately, however, the problem may simply have been that he was unable to explain *how* sugar caused all of these problems. I believe the answer is fructose. In Part II, I will explain why.

THE PRICE OF SUGAR: FRUCTOSE, URIC ACID, AND YOUR HEALTH

CHAPTER 4

SIGNS OF TROUBLE

Fructose and Metabolic Syndrome

Metabolic syndrome. This ominous phrase sounds like the title of a science fiction movie. Unfortunately, metabolic syndrome is not the product of a screenwriter's imagination. It is a very real health menace.

Metabolic syndrome is not a disease. Rather, it's a constellation of five "signs," which is the term doctors use for phenomena that we observe in patients. More than one in four American adults has metabolic syndrome. I have devoted an entire chapter to it because eating a high-fructose diet worsens all aspects of metabolic syndrome, which we know to be a major threat to human health. For example, having metabolic syndrome doubles your odds of suffering a heart attack and increases by fivefold your chances of developing type 2 diabetes. Clearly, it is in your interest to avoid developing metabolic syndrome—and your smartest step toward that goal is to consume less fructose.

In the past few chapters, I explained that the growing consumption of table sugar, high-fructose corn syrup

(HFCS), and other sources of fructose has accompanied a rising rate of obesity and an overall decline in health in the United States and other countries. Until a century or so ago, sugar was an exotic ingredient that only the wealthy could afford. Today, sweet foods and beverages are staples of the American diet. As sugar intake grew, waistlines expanded, and once-rare conditions such as cardiovascular disease and type 2 diabetes became the leading causes of death and disability.

Because fructose is a major component of sugar, does it mean the case against this sweetener is closed? Not quite.

After all, how do we know that the growing dominance of sugar in our diets deserves so much blame for America's burgeoning weight problems and the rapid rise of formerly obscure diseases? Epidemiological studies provide us with powerful clues, but two trends occurring at the same time do not necessarily indicate that one caused the other. By that logic, you could blame the rise of obesity in the United States on the discovery of electricity. Think about it: Didn't electrical current make possible televisions, computers, the Internet, and countless other inventions that increase the amount of time we spend sitting around instead of burning calories through exercise and manual labor?

Furthermore, a cynic might wonder: We're bombarded with scary headlines about health threats in newspapers that often turn out to be false alarms. How do we know that scientists won't discover next year that fructose really isn't so bad after all?

To be sure, the recent past offers striking examples of associations between dietary habits and disease that initially caused worry, yet did not stand up to closer scrutiny. For example, studies in the 1970s and 1980s suggested that drinking coffee causes breast and pancreatic cancers. Yet when scientists examined the link more closely, it disappeared, proving coffee to be innocent. Some research today hints that coffee may actually lower the risk for certain types of cancer (colorectal cancer in particular), as well as type 2 diabetes and Parkinson's disease. (What's more, as I'll explain in a later chapter, drinking coffee may afford some protection against harmful changes that occur in the body when you consume fructose.)

It's also fair to ask another question: Why focus on fructose as the culprit? Remember, table sugar and HFCS are made up of a combination of two simple sugars, fructose and glucose. How do we know that glucose isn't the real problem? This is an important point to consider, because starchy carbohydrates such as bread, pasta, white rice, and potatoes break down to glucose during digestion. Low-carbohydrate diets banish starch from the menu because it causes blood glucose levels to rise.

As I will explain in this chapter, we have powerful direct evidence to show that consuming too much fructose-rich sugar and HFCS causes the toxic brew of conditions known as metabolic syndrome. Moreover, this same body of research suggests that starchy foods do *not* induce metabolic syndrome.

In Part III, I am going to show you how a diet that limits your exposure to fructose and certain other food elements can protect you from developing metabolic syndrome. But first, let's take a closer look at fructose's role in triggering this mysterious complex.

What Is Metabolic Syndrome?

Though metabolic syndrome has become a hot topic in medicine in recent years, the concept is hardly new. More than 80 years ago, a Swedish doctor named Eskil Kylin noticed that a growing number of his patients with elevated blood pressure also had high blood levels of glucose. What's more, they tended to have high blood levels of a compound called uric acid. Dr. Kylin described this syndrome in an article he wrote for a German medical journal in 1923. (*Syndrome* is the term used in medicine to describe a group of signs and symptoms that often occur together.)

Meanwhile, throughout the first half of the 20th century, scientists gradually began to realize that being overweight was not simply a cosmetic concern. Obese people, it became clear, tend to develop diabetes and other disorders and to die prematurely. The view that excess body fat was a serious risk factor for disease gathered steam over the years. Finally, in 1988, Stanford University physician and researcher Gerald Reaven, MD, introduced the idea that obese people often have insulin resistance, elevated blood fats, and certain other conditions that increase the risk for diabetes and heart disease. Dr. Reaven called this collection of symptoms syndrome X.

Syndrome X has undergone several name changes over the years (see "By Any Other Name" on page 57). Today, most doctors call it metabolic syndrome. There is no universal definition of metabolic syndrome, because various medical societies and public health organizations have come up with their own interpretation of which conditions it should include. In 2005, the American Heart Association

---

BY ANY OTHER NAME

Since Gerald Reaven, MD, identified syndrome X in the 1980s, the condition we know as metabolic syndrome has gone by a number of different names, including:

- Reaven's syndrome
- Insulin resistance syndrome
- The Deadly Quartet—a reference to obesity, insulin resistance, high triglycerides, and high blood pressure
- CHAOS, an acronym for coronary artery disease, hypertension, adult-onset diabetes, and obesity)
- Diabesity

(AHA) and the National Heart, Lung, and Blood Institute (NHLBI) established a widely accepted set of guidelines.

The Five Signs of Metabolic Syndrome

Do you have metabolic syndrome? Give yourself one point for each of the following five clinical features that you fulfill. If you score at least three points, then you have metabolic syndrome.

Abdominal obesity. Being overweight is unhealthy, no matter where you carry your excess flab. But fat tissue in and around the abdomen—better known as a spare tire, love handles, or a beer belly—is especially bad for your health. Studies show that people who have the so-called apple silhouette are at an unusually high risk for heart disease, type 2 diabetes, elevated blood fats, and high blood pressure. In fact, their risk for these medical conditions is greater than that of people who are clearly overweight but who carry their extra baggage about the hips (known as a pear shape).

According to the guidelines established by the AHA and NHLBI, you have abdominal obesity if your waist circumference meets these criteria.

- Men: 40 inches or larger

- Women: 35 inches or larger

To measure your waist circumference, wrap a tape measure around your bare abdomen just above the hipbone. The tape should be snug, but not so tight that it squeezes your skin. Take a deep breath, exhale, and measure your waist.

Elevated triglycerides. Most of the fat in food, like most of the fat that pads your body, comes in the form of triglycerides. When you eat more calories than you burn off through physical activity, your liver converts the excess fuel into triglycerides, which are stored in fat cells for later use as energy. If you eat too much or you don't get enough exercise, fat cells keep filling up with triglycerides, and you turn flabby. (As you will learn later on, your liver produces large amounts of triglycerides when you consume fructose.)

Triglycerides travel throughout your body in your blood. Studies show that people with heart disease and diabetes tend to have elevated blood levels of triglycerides. Doctors measure triglycerides after you have fasted overnight or for at least 8 hours. Add one point to your metabolic syndrome score if:

- Your fasting blood triglycerides are 150 milligrams per deciliter (mg/dl) or higher or

- You take medication to lower elevated triglycerides

Low HDL cholesterol. Interestingly, people with metabolic syndrome often have normal levels of total cholesterol and LDL cholesterol, but below-normal levels of HDL cholesterol. As you may know, HDL is often referred to as the "good" cholesterol. Unlike LDL cholesterol, which contributes to the formation of blockages in the arteries, HDL carries cholesterol away from the arteries and back to the liver, which disposes of it. That's why high levels of HDL protect against cardiovascular disease, while low levels encourage atherosclerosis, or the narrowing of arteries that precedes most heart attacks and strokes.

Add one point to your metabolic syndrome score if you meet the following criteria.

- Men: Your HDL is lower than 40 mg/dl

- Women: Your HDL is lower than 50 mg/dl or

- You take medication to increase your HDL level

High blood pressure. Blood pressure refers to the amount of force that blood exerts against the walls of your blood vessels as it circulates throughout your body. A blood pressure reading consists of two numbers that form a fraction, such as 120/75. The first number, called systolic pressure, reflects the force exerted as the heart contracts; the second number, diastolic pressure, indicates the force exerted as the heart relaxes. Blood pressure is measured in millimeters of mercury, abbreviated as mm Hg.

Normally, we diagnose high blood pressure, or hypertension, when a patient's systolic blood pressure is 140 mm Hg or higher, or his or her diastolic blood pressure is 90 mm Hg or higher, or both systolic and diastolic pressures are elevated. Recent studies have made clear that prehypertension—that is, blood pressure that's high but still in the range of what we consider normal—increases the risk for heart disease, too. For this reason, the AHA's guidelines for diagnosing metabolic syndrome use this slightly lower standard for blood pressure.

Add one point to your metabolic syndrome score if:

- Your systolic pressure (the top number) is 130 mm Hg or greater and/or

- Your diastolic pressure (the bottom number) is 85 mm Hg or greater or

- You take medication to treat high blood pressure

Elevated blood glucose. Carbohydrates in food break down into glucose or other sugars before reaching the bloodstream, providing the body with its main source of fuel. In a condition called insulin resistance, which precedes type 2 diabetes, cells aren't able to absorb glucose from the blood. Chronically elevated blood glucose is a sign of insulin resistance and can lead to diabetes complications, such as blindness and nerve damage.

Doctors measure levels of glucose in the blood after you have fasted overnight or for at least 8 hours. Add one point to your metabolic syndrome score if:

- Your fasting blood glucose is 100 mg/dl or higher or

- You take medication to lower blood glucose

The New Metabolic Menace

There has been a disturbing increase in the incidence of metabolic syndrome in the United States over the past generation, as I mentioned in Chapter 1. At present, at least 27 percent of Americans have three or more of the symptoms that make up this deadly syndrome. Some experts believe the actual percentage of Americans with metabolic syndrome is much higher.

Metabolic syndrome does not have a single cause. Likewise, the individual components of metabolic syndrome can be induced by a variety of factors, including genetics, physical activity, and alcohol consumption. What's more, there is a great deal of controversy about whether metabolic syndrome is a useful medical diagnosis. Some doctors believe that knowing a patient has this cluster of conditions can help guide treatment decisions. Yet others say that metabolic syndrome is no greater than the sum of its parts—that you still need to treat each individual condition to lower a patient's risk for heart disease or diabetes.

TWO MORE TO WATCH FOR

If you have metabolic syndrome, there is a good chance that you have two additional risk factors for heart disease and other conditions. They are:

"Sticky" blood. People with metabolic syndrome often have viscous or sticky blood, which forms clots easily. Blood clots can block arteries, resulting in heart attacks and other circulatory problems. To test blood's clotting capacity, doctors measure levels of proteins called plasminogen activator inhibitor-1 and fibrinogen.

Chronic inflammation. Chronic, low-grade inflammation has been implicated in a number of diseases. Doctors check for systemic inflammation by measuring blood levels of C-reactive protein.

This much is not open to debate: Consuming sugar can trigger all of the conditions that make up metabolic syndrome. And the element in sugar that contributes to weight gain, raises blood pressure, elevates blood fats, and causes other dangerous symptoms appears to be fructose.

While epidemiological studies provide clues that sugar and fructose may cause metabolic syndrome, experimental studies allow us to declare them guilty. Scientists have compared the health effects of consuming sugar versus other forms of carbohydrate—namely, starch—in humans and animals. The results of these studies can be summed up by the following observations.

- Sugar (and HFCS) contains fructose and glucose. Studies show that consuming large amounts of sugar produces most symptoms of metabolic syndrome. This suggests that either fructose or glucose is the culprit.

- Starch breaks down into glucose during digestion. Studies show that high-starch diets do not produce symptoms of metabolic syndrome. This suggests that glucose is not the culprit.

- Studies directly comparing fructose and glucose show that fructose produces symptoms of metabolic syndrome, while glucose generally does not.

When I present my diet in Chapter 11, you'll see how understanding these distinctions can allow you to make targeted, specific changes to your daily menu that will help prevent or minimize elements of metabolic syndrome, including weight gain. If losing weight is your main health goal, then reducing your fructose intake is a critical step. Eliminating sources of this sweetener from your diet will help you to stop overeating, control your appetite, and prevent metabolic changes that cause you to build up excess fat.

I'll explain how fructose causes stubborn weight gain over the next few chapters. For now, it's important to mention two points about obesity as it relates to metabolic syndrome.

- Simply being overweight is an important health concern, but excess body fat is considerably more dangerous to your overall well-being if you have other conditions of metabolic syndrome, too.

- You needn't be overweight or obese to have metabolic syndrome. If you exercise regularly, for example, you may be keeping your body fat under control. But if you're also eating a high-fructose diet, you may develop high blood pressure, insulin resistance, and other conditions of metabolic syndrome without realizing it.

In other words, if you're overloading your body with fructose, you may be slowly raising your risk for heart disease and diabetes, independent of any effect that sugar is having on your waistline. Furthermore, as you will soon see, studies show that broadly cutting back on all carbohydrates, as many popular diets recommend, may not be necessary. I believe the best approach is to simply target the true villain: fructose.

A Starch Contrast

The universal fear of all fats that gripped many health-conscious Americans for several decades has been replaced by carbo-phobia. Yet laboratory studies suggest that reducing your intake of sugar and other sources of fructose is the most important step toward preventing metabolic syndrome—far more important than eliminating starchy foods, as low-carbohydrate diets recommend.

Some of the earliest scientific evidence to offer direct proof that eating sweets causes symptoms of metabolic syndrome comes from experiments conducted in the 1960s and 1970s by British physician and scientist John Yudkin, MD, whose antisugar crusade I described in the previous chapter. In a number of studies, Dr. Yudkin and his colleagues compared the effects of feeding high-sugar and high-starch diets to human subjects. Inevitably, his research showed that the former is the greater health threat.

For example, Dr. Yudkin knew from several earlier population studies that people who eat a lot of sugar tend to have low levels of heart-protective HDL cholesterol in their blood. To determine whether the link between eating sugar and low HDL was real, Dr. Yudkin and several other researchers at Queen Elizabeth College in London asked 14 young men to eat a special diet. Normally, the men consumed about 115 grams of sugar daily, on average, which was typical in the United Kingdom at the time. Dr. Yudkin asked them to eat very little starch, while increasing their sugar intake to 252 grams daily, the equivalent of about 60 teaspoons.

That may sound like a lot of sugar, but many heavy consumers ingest at least that much sugar every day—and I'm not just talking about teenagers, either. For instance, Mountain Dew soda—one of the sweeter-tasting soft drinks on the market—is a favorite among computer programmers, who guzzle bottle after bottle while writing code. I know of one programmer who claims that he drinks 2 liters of Mountain Dew per day. That works out to about 59 teaspoons of sugar. (Mountain Dew, like many other brands of soda, contains large amounts of caffeine. As I'll explain in a later chapter, fructose actually raises levels of another compound in the body that mimics caffeine.)

Two weeks into Dr. Yudkin's high-sugar diet, blood tests revealed an alarming trend among the young men: While filling up on sweets, their blood concentrations of HDL cholesterol plummeted. At the study's outset, the average HDL among the participants had been a healthy 50 mg/dl. But 14 days of heavy sugar consumption dropped the typical HDL level to 41 mg/dl. That is perilously close to the minimum benchmark for males, which is 40 mg/dl.

For the second part of his study, Dr. Yudkin asked a group of 26 heavy sugar eaters to cut back on sweet foods for 3 weeks. While their HDL levels didn't change much, eating less sugar appeared to confer another benefit: The study participants' triglyceride levels dropped by 21 percent, on average.

Several later studies failed to confirm Dr. Yudkin's finding that eating fructose has a serious effect on triglycerides. Many scientists remained unconvinced that fructose consistently raised these blood fats until 2000, with the publication of a study in the *American Journal of Clinical Nutrition*. John Bantle, MD, of the University of Minnesota and his team recruited 2 dozen healthy men and women and asked them to follow a high-fructose diet for 6 weeks.

The diet was designed to ensure that the study subjects would be getting 17 percent of their calories from fructose—well within the range for heavy consumers of sugary foods and beverages. Based on government data, Dr. Bantle estimated that up to 27 million Americans consume at least this much fructose.

Next, Dr. Bantle asked the study participants to switch to a very low-fructose diet for 6 weeks. They gave blood samples once a week while on both diets. At the end of the study, the subjects' blood samples showed signs of trouble, at least among the men: Compared with the low-fructose diet, the high-fructose diet caused their triglycerides to shoot up 32 percent. It wasn't clear why the women in Dr. Bantle's study didn't experience a spike in triglyceride levels (though I will describe one possible explanation in a later chapter). Subsequent studies, however, have shown an increase in triglycerides among women who eat a high-fructose diet.

More recent research suggests that consuming a very high-fructose diet over a shorter period can have an even worse effect on triglycerides and cause other metabolic changes that raise the risk for heart disease, especially in people who are overweight. This same research found no ill effects from consuming a high-glucose diet.

Nutrition researcher Peter J. Havel, PhD, of the University of California at Davis and his colleagues asked a group of 13 overweight or obese adults to consume high-fructose beverages every day for 10 weeks. A second group of volunteers drank high-glucose beverages for the same period. The drinks provided 25 percent of the calories that each subject would normally require. Within just 2 weeks, triglyceride levels had soared by 212 percent, on average, among the volunteers given the high-fructose beverages. Meanwhile, tri-glycerides *dropped* among those consuming high-glucose drinks.

Furthermore, the high-fructose beverages—but not the high-glucose drinks—worsened other risk factors for heart disease and other conditions linked to metabolic syndrome. Among the study findings:

- Dr. Havel's team used computed tomography scans to show that abdominal fat increased by nearly 8 percent, on average, in the volunteers given the high-fructose beverages. As I explained earlier in this chapter, abdominal fat is the worst kind, because it raises the risk for heart attack, type 2 diabetes, and other conditions.

- Upon analysis of the volunteers' blood samples, Dr. Havel detected high levels of intracellular adhesion molecule 1, which promotes inflammation in the arteries by causing white blood cells to attach to the arterial lining. As I have noted, many authorities consider chronic low-grade inflammation to be a component of metabolic syndrome. There is no longer any doubt that turning up the heat in the arteries helps to trigger heart attack. (I'll talk more about how a high-fructose diet promotes chronic inflammation in later chapters.)

- Dr. Havel determined that people who consumed high-fructose beverages experienced a 17 percent rise, on average,

in LDL cholesterol. Even worse, their blood
levels of oxidized LDL cholesterol—the kind
that seems to clog arteries—shot up by
15 percent. Although it is not a classic sign
of metabolic syndrome, elevated levels of LDL
cholesterol have been linked to an increased
risk for heart attack and stroke.

Because elevated LDL cholesterol and triglycerides, low
HDL cholesterol, weight gain, and chronic inflammation all
contribute to heart disease, a diet that worsens these risk
factors is cause for serious concern. According to experimental data, fructose-rich sugar damages the heart and
other organs in another way: by raising blood pressure.

In one study, Danish researchers placed a group of
overweight people on a diet that included plenty of soda,
fruit juice, and sugary foods. A second group of volunteers
ate sugar-free foods that contained artificial sweeteners.
After 10 weeks, systolic and diastolic blood pressure had
risen among the sugar eaters. Meanwhile, the study participants on the sugar-free diet experienced a drop in blood
pressure. By the end of the study, there were significant

TURNING SUGAR INTO FAT

It may seem odd that eating fructose, which is a carbohydrate, raises levels
of a fat. But your body is constantly converting one compound into another to
suit its needs. In this case, the transformation occurs in the liver, where most
fructose ends up after a meal. The sugar is processed by an enzyme known as
fructokinase, which breaks down fructose into smaller components. Your
body uses these smaller parts to make either glycogen (the form glucose takes
when it is stored) or triglycerides.

differences in the blood pressure readings of the two groups—6.9 mm Hg systolic, 5.3 mm Hg diastolic.

In the next chapter, I'll talk more about the close link between fructose and a compound in the blood that appears to raise blood pressure and cause other destructive metabolic changes.

Further Lessons from the Lab: Fructose and Insulin Resistance

Elevated blood glucose is one of the key elements of metabolic syndrome that I have not yet discussed in this chapter. A single serving of fructose does not cause your blood glucose level to rise. End of story, right?

Unfortunately, that's far from true. If you consume a high-fructose diet, you could develop the condition known as insulin resistance. As I noted earlier, insulin resistance causes chronically elevated blood glucose. Left untreated, high blood glucose poses a serious threat to your health.

When Dr. Reaven identified the cluster of symptoms he called syndrome X in the 1980s, he believed that insulin resistance was the key underlying problem. In fact, for a time, syndrome X came to be known as insulin resistance syndrome, a phrase that some scientists still use.

Insulin resistance causes type 2 diabetes, which has reached epidemic levels in the United States and many parts of the world. The condition also raises the risk for heart disease. People who develop insulin resistance tend to be overweight; likewise, people who put on too many pounds are more likely to develop insulin resistance. A great deal of powerful scientific evidence suggests that fructose may be the link between obesity and insulin resistance.

To be fair, some research casts doubt on this theory. In one 2006 study, for instance, Swiss scientists asked a group of male volunteers to take a fructose supplement at every meal for a month. None of the men developed insulin resistance. Other studies suggest that fructose may cause only cells in the liver and fat tissue to become insulin resistant, without having any effect on the cells in muscle tissue.

A closer look at these studies reveals potential reasons for their failure to identify a link between fructose and insulin resistance.

- Most of these studies lasted a month or less, so they show only that *acute* fructose ingestion— that is, over a short period—does not cause insulin resistance. They don't give any indication whether *chronic*, long-term fructose consumption—like what you would experience from a lifetime of eating and drinking sugary foods and beverages—causes insulin resistance. Yet we know from studies that feeding a low dose of fructose to laboratory rats every day for an extended period— 15 months—causes them to become insulin resistant.

- It's not surprising that some studies found only that fructose caused insulin resistance in liver and fat cells. These cells have the highest levels of fructokinase, or fructose enzymes, which allows the body to process fructose. (You will be reading much more about the damaging effects of this enzyme in the pages to come.) If these studies had lasted longer, I suspect they would have shown that a high-fructose diet causes full-blown insulin resistance, among other conditions of metabolic syndrome. In the study by Dr. Havel that I mentioned earlier, the volunteers who consumed fructose-sweetened beverages for 10 weeks showed elevated insulin levels, indicating that their cells were resisting the hormone's effects— an early sign of diabetes. The volunteers who drank glucose-sweetened beverages did not develop insulin resistance.

- The studies showing no effect from high-fructose diets tended to have healthy young people as their subjects. They're more likely to be getting plenty of exercise, which makes cells more sensitive to insulin. In other words, the physical activity could have offset any insulin resistance caused by fructose. These studies *don't* tell us how a high-fructose diet might affect people who—like millions of Americans— may already be mildly insulin resistant because they are sedentary or they have a weight problem. In one study, middle-aged men with elevated insulin levels who followed a diet that derived 15 percent of its calories from fructose developed signs of insulin resistance after 5 weeks, while a similar group who ate a high-starch diet did not. What's truly worrisome about this finding is that many people who consume lots of sugary foods and soft drinks take in that much fructose every day.

A number of other studies have shown that eating a high-fructose diet makes cells resist insulin. For example, Dr. Yudkin found that about one-third of his study subjects who consumed high-sugar diets became insulin resistant. In another especially interesting study, Danish researchers asked seven men to eat their normal diets for 1 week, with an additional 1,000 calories of pure glucose each day. The result? Nothing. Their insulin worked fine. A high intake of glucose had no effect on cells and their ability to use insulin. When the men switched from glucose to 1,000 calories of extra fructose every day, however, the results were much different: Special blood tests showed that the participants' insulin became 25 percent less effective over the course of 1 week.

Our research at the University of Florida further strengthens the theory that sugary foods cause insulin resistance—but bread, potatoes, and other starchy foods do not. We showed this by feeding high-carbohydrate diets to two groups of laboratory rats. One group received their carbohydrates in the form of fructose, while the other got their carbs from starch, which breaks down to glucose (also called dextrose) in the body. Both groups received the same amount of food each day, as measured in calories.

After a month, we weighed and evaluated the rats. All of them had gained weight, regardless of what they ate. Because they were given the same amount of food, we did not expect to see any difference in weight. Nevertheless, the rats fed fructose gained slightly more weight than those fed starch. From a statistical standpoint, the difference was not significant. Had the study gone on longer, however, the rats eating fructose all day might have gained considerably more weight than those eating starch.

There was no ambiguity when we analyzed the rats'

blood. The fructose-fed rats had sky-high triglycerides—four times higher than their starch-eating counterparts.

When we checked the rats' insulin levels, we discovered something else just as provocative. Dietary starch had no effect on insulin; the rats eating dextrose showed no change in their insulin levels after 4 weeks. By comparison, insulin levels jumped dramatically among the rats that were eating a high-fructose diet. Their blood concentration of insulin was nearly twice as high, on average, as in the rats given dextrose.

High insulin levels, a condition known as hyperinsulinemia, indicate that body tissue is not able to use the hormone properly. In other words, eating fructose made the rats insulin resistant—yet eating glucose did not. This suggests that the rise in blood glucose that occurs when you eat a lot of starchy foods isn't necessarily harmful. What really matters is whether the cells in the body's tissue become resistant to insulin's effects. This is what happens when you gain weight, and it's what causes type 2 diabetes. The science is clear on this point: Neither high glucose intake nor high blood glucose levels cause insulin resistance.

On the other hand, our research suggests that eating a high-fructose diet *does* cause insulin resistance—and I believe we know why. Our experiment with laboratory rats, like other studies involving humans, shows that consuming fructose also raises blood levels of uric acid. As you may recall, the Swedish physician Eskil Kylin included elevated uric acid in the troika of common symptoms that he first described in the 1920s.

In the next chapter, you will learn why uric acid is one of the most critical, and critically misunderstood, compounds in the human body. Uric acid, which rises when you eat a diet rich in fructose and certain other foods, appears to increase the risk for weight gain and other conditions of metabolic syndrome. Simply put, if your uric acid rises, your health is probably in danger.

Over the past half-century, we have learned to avoid eating too much saturated fat for fear of raising blood cholesterol. As I'm about to show, avoiding fructose to keep your uric acid under control could be a lifesaver, too.

CHAPTER 5

THE ACID TEST

Fructose and the Return of an Old Threat

Is there something your doctor isn't telling you?

If you have been eating the typical American diet, you have probably been consuming a great deal of fructose—in which case, you may have high levels of a substance called uric acid in your blood. Knowing whether or not you have elevated uric acid could help your physician predict if you are going to gain weight, have a heart attack, or develop diabetes—and allow him or her to develop a treatment plan that could help you avoid these fates.

Fortunately, there is a simple, inexpensive blood test to measure uric acid. In fact, it has been around for years.

Unfortunately, your doctor probably doesn't use it.

How could this be? After all, your physician dutifully checks your blood for a long list of other disease markers when you get an annual physical exam. There are the usual suspects, including cholesterol, triglycerides, and fasting blood glucose, as well as liver enzymes, electrolytes, and calcium. In recent years, some physicians have begun testing for a new generation of blood elements that have been linked to heart disease, such as fibrinogen, a protein that causes blood to clot, and C-reactive protein, a marker of low-grade arterial inflammation.

All of this information helps your doctor determine what kind of shape you are in and predict what health concerns might be around the corner. Yet few doctors bother to check their patients' blood levels of uric acid, a common substance that can provide valuable insight into your general well-being. If you have high uric acid, for example, you could be on your way to developing metabolic syndrome, the deadly quintet of conditions I described in the previous chapter.

Many health-conscious people can recite their cholesterol, blood pressure, and other vital statistics from memory. Why don't you know your uric acid level?

There are several reasons that your doctor probably does not measure uric acid as part of a physical exam. No major medical or health organization currently recommends routine screening for elevated uric acid. Medical schools teach physicians-in-training that high levels of this compound increase the risk for just a few medical conditions, none life threatening or common enough to warrant broad-based testing.

Now emerging scientific evidence strongly suggests that if uric acid is too high, serious health problems lie ahead. For example, a 2007 study of more than 8,500 people published in the *American Journal of Medicine (AJM)* found that 70 percent of those with very high uric acid levels had metabolic syndrome. In another 2007 study that appeared in the journal *Circulation*, researchers showed that children and adolescents with the highest levels of uric acid were nearly 15 times more likely than kids with low uric acid to have metabolic syndrome.

As you will read later in these pages, people with high uric acid often end up gaining substantial amounts of weight. But even if you are not presently overweight, elevated uric acid may be harming your health in other ways. In the *AJM* study, nearly 60 percent of people who had high uric acid—but were normal in size—had other conditions of metabolic syndrome, such as high blood pressure or insulin resistance.

Uric acid is controversial. Not all scientists believe that it's an important risk factor for obesity and metabolic syndrome. There are those who say that uric acid is benign and poses no danger. Others argue that uric acid is actually beneficial.

As I will show you in this chapter, mounting research indicates that people who have high uric acid levels are more likely to become overweight or obese and develop heart disease, type 2 diabetes, and other leading killers. Because uric

---

GETTING YOUR URIC ACID TESTED

In Chapter 11, I am going to describe a diet that will help to lower your uric acid. You can track your weight loss on the bathroom scale, but to determine whether you are successfully lowering your uric acid—which will help you to maintain weight loss and protect against heart disease, diabetes, and other serious conditions—I recommend getting a baseline measurement and a follow-up test 1 to 2 months after you begin the Low-Fructose Diet.

Any blood lab can measure your uric acid. You should fast for at least 4 hours before the test, which is performed by drawing a small blood sample from a vein. Your doctor may also advise you to stop taking certain medications beforehand. Use the following benchmarks as goals.

- For men: 5.5 mg/dl or lower
- For women: 5.0 mg/dl or lower

acid rises when you eat fructose, as well as certain other foods, this means an alarming number of Americans could be at risk.

Ironically, up until the early 1980s, a uric acid assay was a component of the standard blood panel that doctors used for health screening. I predict that one day in the near future, uric acid screening will once again be a standard part of routine physical exams. But why wait? I believe you should have your uric acid checked *now* along with your cholesterol, blood glucose, and other disease risk factors. In this chapter, I'll explain why.

What Is Uric Acid?

The cells that make up every piece of tissue in your body have a limited life span. As they naturally die off, they break down into smaller parts. The uric acid story begins with DNA, the nucleic acid that serves as the genetic blueprint for every cell in your body, and RNA, the messenger that carries out DNA's instructions.

As old cells break down, DNA and RNA degrade into smaller parts, including components called purines. Enzymes convert purines into a substance called xanthine. Over time, xanthine degrades further into uric acid. Your body also produces uric acid as it burns adenosine triphosphate (ATP), an organic compound in cells that plays a vital role in producing energy.

All animals have uric acid in their blood. Most mammals, fish, and amphibians show very low levels, because they possess an enzyme that converts uric acid into another substance, called allantoin. Humans evolved without this enzyme, known as uricase, so we tend to have relatively high uric acid levels. So, too, do birds and reptiles. Just two other types of mammals lack uricase: the great and lesser apes (such as chimpanzees, gibbons, gorillas, and orang-utans), and some New World monkeys.

Although humans evolved with relatively high uric acid, your grandparents or great-grandparents probably had lower levels than you do. Among Americans, the typical uric acid level has risen significantly since the early half of the 20th century. In the 1920s, for example, the average uric acid level among adult males in the United States was about 3.5 milli-grams per deciliter of blood (abbreviated as mg/dl). More recent studies, using a different type of test, show a gradual increase in uric acid since the early 1950s. By 1980, typical uric acid levels in adult males climbed into the range of 6.0 to 6.5 mg/dl. Keeping in mind that fructose raises uric acid, and that we consume more of this sugar today than at any other time in history, these figures are probably even higher now.

Just as cholesterol levels vary greatly from one person to another, so do uric acid levels, which typically fall some-where between 3.0 and 8.0 mg/dl in humans. (They can dip as low as 2 mg/dl and rise as high as 15 mg/dl.) Chil-dren tend to have low concentrations, usually less than 5 mg/dl, but this changes during puberty—at least among males. Females maintain relatively low uric acid levels during the first few decades of adulthood. They appear to gain this protection because the hormone estrogen in-creases the amount of uric acid they eliminate in urine.

It is possible that some of the difference between males and females may simply be chalked up to men eating more foods that elevate uric acid. As you will soon see, diet has a major impact on how much of this compound is in your blood. Once women reach menopause, though, their uric acid levels climb. Among males and females over age 50, uric acid concentrations are similar.

THE BEER BELLY AND URIC ACID

If you love lager, ale, or other frothy libations, then you may carry with you visual proof in the form of a beer belly. A paunchy midsection doesn't flatter anyone's appearance, and in addition, it may serve as a strong indicator that you are developing serious metabolic problems. In particular, a beer belly may signal that you already have metabolic syndrome and that your uric acid levels are too high.

Alcohol not only causes your body to produce uric acid, it also blocks the kidneys from excreting the compound. In theory, this means that any type of alcoholic beverage should cause hyperuricemia, or elevated uric acid levels. Beer seems to have an unusually strong effect on uric acid.

We know, for example, that drinking beer increases the risk for gout—a disease caused by elevated uric acid—more than other forms of alcohol. Massachusetts General Hospital rheumatologist Hyon K. Choi, MD, and several colleagues found that men who drink two or more beers per day were 2.5 times more likely to develop gout than men who abstained. By contrast, Dr. Choi found that several glasses of spirits raised the risk of gout by just 1.6 times, while a moderate amount of wine had no effect at all.

Beer may raise uric acid levels more than other types of alcoholic beverages because it is a rich source of guanosine, the type of purine that is most readily absorbed by the body. Remember, purines break down into uric acid, so it's not surprising that the amber brew has a greater impact on uric acid levels than other forms of alcohol.

I think of the beer belly as a *forme fruste* (pronounced form FROOST) of metabolic syndrome, which is the term we use in medicine for an incomplete or unusual form of a disease. In this case, flab hanging over your belt buckle may be early evidence of worse things to come. Along with excess abdominal fat, many people with beer bellies have other conditions of metabolic syndrome, particularly elevated triglycerides and high blood pressure. Although many beer devotees don't want to hear this, you might be better off satisfying a taste for an occasional alcoholic beverage with a glass of Merlot or Chardonnay instead.

Not by Fructose Alone

Fructose increases uric acid levels through a complex process that causes cells to burn up their ATP rapidly. As you will learn in the next chapter, if you eat a diet rich in foods that contain fructose, your body will become highly efficient at producing uric acid. Over time, your body becomes "primed" to churn out large amounts of uric acid, even if you consume just a small serving of sugar, high-fructose corn syrup, or any other source of fructose.

To be sure, uric acid levels are greatly influenced by your diet and can fluctuate wildly, depending on what you eat. Sweet foods are not the only ones that increase uric acid. As you will recall, the naturally occurring uric acid in your body is formed from organic compounds called purines, which are produced as your body breaks down and eliminates old cells. Certain foods contain purines, too— sometimes at very high levels. Eating purine-rich foods can also raise uric acid.

Fortunately, many of the worst offenders are probably not atop your list of favorite foods, unless you have a particular fondness for liver, brains, kidneys, and other organ meats, which have some of the highest purine levels. Shellfish (such as shrimp and lobster) and certain dark-fleshed fish (such as anchovies, herring, sardines, and mackerel) are high in purines, too, while red meats have more modest levels. Some vegetables contain rather large amounts of purines, though research suggests that they have little if any effect on uric acid. Each year, Americans drink about 6 billion gallons of another rich source of purines: beer.

Eating fewer purine-rich foods can help you to main-

URIC ACID, LEAD POISONING, AND THE FALL OF THE ROMAN EMPIRE

Eating too much food that contains fructose and purines is not the only way to develop elevated uric acid. Consuming small quantities of lead will have the same effect, because the presence of this heavy metal in the body prevents the kidneys from passing uric acid in the urine.

While most diets today do not contain appreciable amounts of lead, that hasn't been the case throughout history. In fact, elevated uric acid from lead contamination may have been responsible for several epidemics over the centuries.

For example, the form of arthritis known as gout—which is caused by high uric acid levels—was rampant among the upper class during the Roman Empire. Indeed, many of the Roman emperors had the condition. A favorite pastime among wealthy Romans of the day was drinking wine sweetened with a syrup called sapa, which was made from crushed grapes simmered in lead pots. Sapa was sometimes added to certain foods, too.

Doctors long ago identified a form of gout, known as saturnine gout, caused by lead contamination. But aching joints (especially in the big toe) may not have been the only health woe suffered by ancient Roman wine lovers. Increased lead exposure can result in anemia, abdominal pain, mental disturbances, and neurological disorders. Environmental chemist Jerome Nriagu has suggested that lead intoxication may have contributed to the fall of the Roman Empire.

A second major outbreak of gout occurred during the 18th and 19th centuries in England, a time when the British aristocracy had developed a taste for port that had been shipped overseas in lead-lined casks. Historians have noted that this more recent gout epidemic was not limited to the upper class; many

---

tain safe uric acid levels. I'll give you a complete list of foods to avoid or eat in moderation in Chapter 11. I'll also show you why adding certain foods—especially low-fat milk and other dairy products—can help you lower uric acid.

Uric Acid and Your Weight

Eating too much fructose causes you to gain weight and interferes with your ability to lose weight, even if you attempt to cut calories. I'll describe the many different ways that fructose promotes weight gain in the next chapter. As I'll explain here, a high-fructose diet creates persistently ele-

artisans and artists—who were exposed to lead while making pottery, blowing glass, and painting—developed the disease, too. Plumbers, who spent much of their time repairing lead pipes, also appear to have been susceptible. (In fact, "plumbism" is the word for lead intoxication.)

During this era, some doctors in England noted that chronic lead ingestion not only increased uric acid levels but also was associated with high blood pressure and kidney disease. Did high uric acid cause these diseases? It's now well established that exposure to even low lead levels can induce hypertension in both laboratory animals and humans. Experiments by my group at the University of Florida show that we can reduce lead-induced high blood pressure in rats by giving them drugs that lower uric acid. Furthermore, we have found that ingesting lead causes the same kinds of changes in the kidneys that we see in humans and lab rats with high uric acid.

In the United States, the typical blood level of lead has dropped dramatically since the 1970s, probably due to removal of the metal from gasoline, paint, and other products, as well as stricter laws regarding exposure in the workplace. Still, worries about lead exposure have resurfaced in recent years because of concerns about high levels in imported products ranging from toys to toothpaste. Worrisome research suggests that even low levels of lead exposure over the long term can increase the risk for heart disease and other health problems. Clearly, we have much to learn about this issue, but I believe it's possible that exposure to lead and our appetites for fructose-sweetened foods may produce similar effects in the body.

vated uric acid, which can have a serious impact on your waistline. Simply stated, the higher your uric acid, the more likely you are to become overweight or obese.

Consider, for example, what Japanese scientists discovered when they examined the link between uric acid and weight gain. For a 2003 study, Osaka University researcher Kazuko Masuo, MD, and his colleagues assembled 433 normal-size men. They weighed each man and then measured his uric acid. Over the next 5 years, Dr. Masuo's team reweighed each man and rechecked his uric acid annually.

By the end of the study, a group of the men had gained

a lot of weight—more than 16 pounds per person, on average. The researchers also identified a subset of the men who had gained little or no weight. A comparison of the uric acid levels of the two groups at the start of the 5-year study produced a striking difference: Among those who had gained weight, uric acid was nearly 30 percent higher. What's more, as these men put on more pounds, their uric acid levels continued to climb, from 5.5 mg/dl to 6.1 mg/dl on average.

This study suggests that having high uric acid makes you vulnerable to putting on weight. How? We can't be certain, but some important clues have recently emerged. For instance, one leading obesity researcher has shown that blocking production of uric acid may be a key to fighting flab.

Rockefeller University molecular geneticist Jeffrey M. Friedman, MD, made a major contribution to the study of obesity in the 1990s when he discovered leptin, a hormone that helps to regulate appetite. More recently, Dr. Friedman and his team showed that mice lacking an enzyme called xanthine oxidoreductase, or XO, don't become fat. In fact, they have 50 percent less fat than mice with XO. What is XO's role in the body? It makes uric acid. This suggests that slowing down production of uric acid might help to prevent the accumulation of excess body fat.

Dr. Friedman's findings build upon some intriguing clues that my colleagues and I have uncovered. We have shown, for example, that feeding rats a high-fructose diet makes them gain weight and causes their uric acid levels to rise. (Interestingly, rats *don't* become fat when they are fed glucose in the form of starch.) When we added a drug called allopurinol to the drinking water of another group of rats, they maintained normal uric acid levels—and didn't gain

SUGAR AND HYPERACTIVITY

Many parents are convinced that eating too much candy or drinking soda gives their children a "sugar buzz," causing them to run amok and misbehave. Some scientists have even speculated that a high-sugar diet contributes to hyperactivity disorders. Most controlled trials have failed to show that consuming sugary foods causes behavior problems in children, however. Yet some research suggests an explanation for the gap between parents' perceptions and the science.

As I have explained, consuming fructose-rich foods causes uric acid to rise. Uric acid is chemically similar to caffeine, a stimulant. Studies show that hyperactive children tend to have high uric acid. Other studies indicate that the amount of uric acid generated by humans following a dose of fructose is highly dependent on the volume and activity of enzymes in the liver known as fructokinase, or fructose enzymes. As such, the amount of uric acid produced by a child after eating a candy bar or gulping down a cola can vary greatly. It's important to note that many soft drinks contain large amounts of caffeine, too. If, indeed, drinking sweetened beverages causes behavior changes, it may be due to the combined effects of fructose and caffeine.

Do fructose and uric acid make children restless and mischievous? To test this theory, psychologists would need to assemble a group of children who appear to become hyperactive after consuming sugar, feed them a large dose of fructose, then measure their uric acid levels. To my knowledge, such a study has not been performed.

weight—while on a high-fructose diet. Allopurinol blocks the formation of uric acid.

As I will explain in the next chapter, uric acid and fructose appear to promote weight gain by acting directly on fat cells, or adipocytes. Our research suggests that even if you are not currently overweight but you consume large amounts of fructose, your fat cells may already be inflamed and experiencing a form of damage called oxidative stress. In other words, long-term exposure to fructose and uric acid seems to turn healthy cells that store the modest amounts of fat necessary for energy into sickly cells that become bloated with excess oxidized fats.

The Gout Connection

You may not have heard of uric acid before picking up this book, but it is hardly a recent discovery. Scientists have been studying, and debating, uric acid for centuries. During the 1800s, some doctors believed that elevated uric acid caused many of the curious new diseases that were becoming more common with each passing year, such as high blood pressure. Others saw uric acid as a kind of all-purpose scourge, responsible for an even wider range of chronic and acute diseases.

With the arrival of the 20th century, however, many researchers eventually shifted their focus to other novel risk factors in the blood, such as cholesterol. Some dismissed uric acid altogether, insisting that it is not a significant health threat. Fortunately, there has been a resurrection of interest in this provocative substance in recent years. Solid research suggests that a rising uric acid level not only plays a key role in weight gain, it also triggers changes in the body that increase the risk for many other conditions of metabolic syndrome. In particular, we now have powerful evidence indicating that elevated uric acid escalates your chances of developing heart disease, the leading cause of death in the United States.

A German pharmacist named Karl W. Scheele discovered uric acid in 1776. Uric acid is just one of many important elements that Scheele identified. In fact, some historians believe that he discovered oxygen, though Joseph Priestley, an English clergyman and chemist, usually gets the credit.

Doctors have known since the 19th century that high blood levels of uric acid can cause gout, an excruciating form of arthritis. Gout was one of the first medical conditions identified by the earliest physicians, dating back to the days of Hippocrates. It occurs when uric acid forms crystals in the joints and surrounding tissues. Any joint can be affected, but about 75 percent of sufferers develop unbearable pain in the big toe. (No one is sure why gout strikes in the big toe so often, but it may be that uric acid crystals form more readily in the cooler blood temperature of body parts farthest from the heart.) Gout patients often describe their joints as becoming so sensitive that they can't bear any pressure. Even the weight of a bedsheet can cause them to writhe in agony.

Physicians long believed gout to be a disease of the upper classes, because only the wealthy could afford to eat the rich foods that raise uric acid. But history shows us that gout became more common and widespread in the United Kingdom and Germany in the 19th century, at the same time that sugar consumption was rising in those countries. (Studies also suggest that the incidence of gout is on the rise in the United States; currently, about 10 million Americans have the disease.)

As gout was causing big toes to throb throughout Victorian England, doctors there began to notice that most people with the disease were overweight. They also seemed to have an unusually high risk for developing the serious emerging medical conditions of the day, such as cardiovascular disease, high blood pressure, diabetes, and kidney disease. Some physicians saw an obvious connection between gout and these other conditions and suspected that uric acid might cause more than sore joints. For example, the British doctor who first described essential hypertension in 1879, Frederick Akbar Mahomed, MD, wrote that people with high blood pressure "frequently belong to gouty families or have themselves suffered from this disease." Dr. Mahomed called uric acid a "blood poison."

A GREATER THREAT?

Some 19th-century physicians believed that uric acid raised blood pressure and caused other conditions of what we now know as metabolic syndrome. Yet at least one doctor saw uric acid as an even greater threat. Alexander Haig, MD, a physician at London's Metropolitan Hospital, wrote a book titled *Uric Acid as a Factor in the Causation of Disease*, which first published in 1892.

Dr. Haig (who was not related to the former US secretary of state of the same name) became interested in uric acid because he suffered frequent migraines. He had tried to cure his headaches with a variety of nostrums and dietary changes, but none worked. Finally, he gave up meat and subsisted primarily on fish and milk. Within months, his headaches had practically disappeared. Dr. Haig concluded that lowering his uric acid by banishing meat from his menu had been his salvation.

But he didn't stop there. In his book, Dr. Haig linked elevated blood levels of uric acid to high blood pressure, diabetes, and gout, as well as anemia, asthma, bronchitis, depression, epilepsy, kidney disease, and rheumatoid arthritis, among other disorders. The reading public was intrigued; the book became very popular and was reissued several times.

Studies conducted during the first half of the 20th century found that the majority of people with gout—70 percent—were obese. Between 50 and 60 percent had hypertension, and half had chronic kidney disease. Most alarming of all, 9 of 10 gout patients eventually developed some form of heart disease, which ultimately killed up to one-quarter of them. One of the key reasons that gout patients suffer from so many other serious medical conditions appears to be that they have too much uric acid in their blood.

Uric Acid and Your Heart

As I explained in the previous chapter, people who consume too much fructose tend to gain weight and develop other conditions of metabolic syndrome. This deadly spectrum of conditions raises your risk for several leading killers, particularly heart disease. We have excellent scientific evidence to suggest that lowering your uric acid could help to control one critical component of metabolic syndrome: high blood pressure.

Consider this: A study in New York City of 8,690 people found that every 1 mg/dl drop in uric acid is equivalent to a 10-point drop in systolic blood pressure—a change that could cut your risk for a heart attack by 32 percent. (This study also showed that 1 mg/dl drop in uric acid is equal to cutting your total cholesterol by 46 mg/dl.)

A great deal of research links uric acid to high blood pressure. In fact, 16 of 17 studies show that people with elevated uric acid are at significantly increased risk for developing essential hypertension, the most common cause of high blood pressure. Further, studies show that people with high blood levels of uric acid are at increased risk for high blood pressure even if they have no other conditions of metabolic syndrome. In one of the largest investigations of its kind, involving 10,000 people, those with high uric acid had double the risk for high blood pressure compared with those with normal uric acid. In some studies, the impact of high uric acid appears to be even greater.

There are several forms of high blood pressure, of which essential hypertension is by far the most common. Your blood pressure may rise with certain drugs or as a side effect of some other condition, such as kidney disease. This rise in blood pressure is known as secondary hypertension, which usually clears up if you switch to a different medication or treat the condition that's causing it.

Essential hypertension accounts for 90 to 95 percent of all cases of high blood pressure. It raises the risk not only for heart attack but also for stroke, heart failure, and kidney disease. The underlying cause of essential hypertension is unknown, making it one of the great mysteries of modern medicine.

I have devoted much of my work as a scientist to exploring the root causes of essential hypertension. My research eventually led me to uric acid. Along with my colleagues, I have conducted a number of studies that persuasively link uric acid to blood pressure.

For example, when Daniel Feig, MD, of Baylor College of Medicine in Houston and I studied a large group of children recently diagnosed with hypertension, we found that 89 percent of them had elevated uric acid (which we defined as 5.5 mg/dl or higher). For comparison, we analyzed the blood of another group of children with normal blood pressure. Not one of them had high uric acid.

Likewise, we looked at children with secondary hypertension—that is, high blood pressure caused by some other disease or a medication—and found that most of them had normal uric acid. The same was true of children with so-called white coat hypertension, which is a rise in blood pressure that's caused by the anxiety of undergoing a medical exam. (The person's blood pressure is normal when measured outside of the clinic.)

Finally, we also considered the potential role of obesity, which is associated with high blood pressure. We compared the weights of the children recently diagnosed with hypertension with those of the children with white coat hypertension (who, remember, have normal uric acid and healthy blood pressure outside a doctor's office). There was no difference: Obesity was just as much a problem in both groups. Taken together, these findings tell us that rising uric acid is not merely a byproduct of high blood pressure or obesity.

Uric Acid and High Blood Pressure: Powerful Evidence

As I have tried to emphasize in the preceding pages, just because two phenomena occur together—such as elevated uric acid and high blood pressure—it does not prove that one causes the other. By this logic, you could assume that a rooster's crow causes the sun to rise. Confirming the theory that elevated uric acid raises blood pressure—which would mean that *reducing* blood levels of uric acid protects against heart disease and stroke—requires rigorous testing.

In science, the gold-standard test for proving a theory is called a double-blind, placebo-controlled trial. In these strictly designed studies, one group of subjects receives a treatment while another group receives a placebo—that is, an empty pill or another nontherapeutic agent that has been designed to look, smell, and taste like the real treatment. Further, neither the subjects nor the scientists conducting the study know who received the active treatment and who received the placebo (which is why it's called a double-blind trial). At the end of such a trial, investigators compare the two groups to determine whether the treatment had any effect. The design of such a study helps us to produce genuine, reliable results by eliminating investigators' biases, the possibility of the outcome simply occurring by chance, and the so-called placebo effect—that is, the phenomenon in which some people experience improvements or changes in their health simply because they *think* they are receiving a beneficial therapy.

The first gold-standard test of whether lowering uric acid improves blood pressure was led by my colleague Dr. Feig. I met Dr. Feig in the fall of 2001, shortly after he arrived as a young assistant professor at Baylor, where I was chief and professor of adult nephrology at the time. Dr. Feig met with me to talk about research and to ask me to act as his mentor. When I learned that he was running one of the largest hypertension clinics for adolescents in Houston, I suggested that we study the role of uric acid in his patients. Dr. Feig and I both believed that hypertension and uric acid were somehow connected, but neither of us was quite prepared for what we discovered.

As I mentioned earlier, Dr. Feig and I had studied a group of adolescents with hypertension and found high uric acid levels in nearly 9 out of 10 of them. Given these dramatic findings, Dr. Feig devised a clinical trial to determine if reducing uric acid would lower blood pressure in these patients. Dr. Feig recruited 30 adolescents (average age 15) who had recently been diagnosed with mild essential hypertension. Most of the young men and women were obese. Dr. Feig gave half of the study subjects the drug allopurinol, which lowers uric acid, with instructions to take the pills twice a day. The other half received placebo pills.

After 4 weeks, Dr. Feig checked the blood pressure of all of the young men and women participating in the study. After a 2-week break, he continued the study by switching the treatments—that is, subjects who had been taking allopurinol now got the placebo pills, while the young people who had been taking placebo pills now got uric acid–lowering allopurinol. After another 4 weeks, Dr. Feig measured the participants' blood pressure again.

The results of the study, which were published in the *Journal of the American Medical Association* in 2008, were clear and unambiguous. While the young men and women with hypertension were taking allopurinol, their uric acid levels dropped—and so did their blood pressure. The reduction was significant; on average, systolic blood pressure (the top number) dropped 5 mm Hg, while diastolic pressure (the lower number) fell 2.5 mm Hg.

Because blood pressure measurements taken in the clinic are often influenced by the placebo effect, Dr. Feig had the participants wear special monitors that record blood pressure over a 24-hour period. These readings—which are a better predictor of which patients will develop heart disease—showed that lowering uric acid led to even more impressive reductions in blood pressure: 7 mm Hg (systolic) and 4 mm Hg (diastolic). This means that the blood pressure–lowering effect of allopurinol equaled that of most commonly used hypertension medications.

Needless to say, this was an exciting result, because it offered the first solid evidence that lowering elevated uric acid can prevent heart attack, stroke, and other conditions, such as kidney disease. I need to mention a caveat or two, however. This study involved adolescents with mild, recently diagnosed hypertension, so we can't be sure that lowering uric acid will be equally effective in adults, or in patients with longstanding or severe hypertension. It's also possible that the allopurinol lowered blood pressure through a mechanism that does not involve uric acid. Nevertheless, this study provides some of the strongest clinical evidence to date that uric acid is a true risk factor for cardiovascular disease.

Other groups have examined the effects of uric acid on blood pressure, and the results of their investigations support what Dr. Feig and I showed in our study of adolescents with hypertension. For example, a team of Turkish scientists gave allopurinol to a group of volunteers with high uric acid levels (which they defined as 7.0 mg/dl or higher). Lowering uric acid with allopurinol not only reduced the study subjects' blood pressure, it also reduced their levels of C-reactive protein—an indicator of potentially damaging arterial inflammation—and improved their kidney function.

In another study, Egyptian scientists looked at a group of patients with kidney disease who were taking allopurinol. When the allopurinol was removed from their treatment regimens, a subset of the patients—specifically, those who were not taking blood pressure medications called ACE inhibitors—experienced a marked rise in blood pressure. Their kidney function worsened at a faster rate, too. Yet another study by researchers from Hong Kong showed that lowering uric acid slowed the loss of kidney function in patients with kidney disease.

What I find most exciting of all about this groundbreaking research is that it could apply to anyone who wants to improve his or her health. We have compelling evidence that lowering uric acid appears to protect against heart disease and other conditions. But you don't need drugs to get moving in the right direction. Adopting the Low-Fructose Diet, which I describe in Chapter 11, will cause levels of this troublesome compound to drop, too.

What's So Bad About Uric Acid?

Scientists have been trying to explain the cause of essential hypertension for decades. With our sights set on elevated uric acid as an important influence, we are trying to answer a critical question: *How* does uric acid raise blood pressure? Research from our laboratory points to three potential mechanisms that could provide the answer.

Uric acid and nitric oxide. As uric acid spills into the blood after you consume a food or beverage that's high in fructose or purines, it shuts down production of a gas called nitric oxide. Healthy circulation requires blood vessels to expand and contract. To expand blood vessels, endothelial cells that line the blood vessel walls produce nitric oxide. This important gas acts as a messenger, instructing the smooth muscle cells that surround blood ves-

---

NITRIC OXIDE: A NOBEL GAS

Until the mid-1970s, most scientists believed that nitric oxide (NO) was simply a toxic gas found in automobile exhaust and lightning strikes. Then researchers studying chemical "messengers" in the body discovered that NO plays a crucial role in promoting healthy circulation by causing blood vessels to relax.

Initially, most scientists found this theory absurd. After all, beyond the fact that NO is a noxious gas, the molecule itself is a free radical, meaning that it is missing electrons. As a result, NO has the potential to damage healthy tissue in the body as it searches to restore the absent electrons. Still, your body produces small amounts of NO—enough to keep blood vessels open and flowing, but too little to do any damage.

Today, the beneficial role of NO in human health is widely accepted. Three of the scientists who proved its importance in the cardiovascular system won the Nobel Prize in 1998. It's since been established that NO has other important benefits, too.

For example, the knowledge that NO promotes blood flow in the penis allowed drugmakers to develop erectile dysfunction treatments such as Viagra. What's more, recognizing the role of NO explained why nitroglycerin tablets are an effective treatment for people with angina pectoris, or chest pain that occurs when blood flow to the heart is diminished, starving the cardiac muscle of oxygen. The body converts nitroglycerin to nitric oxide, which dilates the coronary arteries, improving the flow of oxygen-rich blood to the heart.

A bit of trivia: As you may know, nitroglycerin is the key ingredient in dynamite. Interestingly, Alfred Nobel invented dynamite and used his wealth to institute the Nobel Prize. Yet according to some accounts, when Nobel developed angina, he refused to take the nitroglycerin pills his doctors prescribed, fearing that they would cause severe headaches.

sels to stop contracting. As uric acid blocks the release of nitric oxide, blood vessels cannot relax and dilate, which raises blood pressure.

Uric acid and angiotensin. In addition to blocking nitric oxide, uric acid raises blood pressure in another way: It stimulates production of a molecule called angiotensin, which causes blood vessels to constrict. In a sense, then, uric acid has the opposite effect of drugs commonly prescribed to treat hypertension called ACE inhibitors. These drugs block the enzymes necessary to form angiotensin. (ACE stands for angiotensin-converting enzyme.) A related class of drugs, known as angiotensin receptor blockers, prevents angiotensin from working properly.

Uric acid and kidney damage. The kidneys play a critical role in regulating the volume of all fluids in the body, including the blood. We have shown that uric acid produces subtle injuries to the kidneys. This damage causes the kidneys to retain sodium, which increases the volume of blood in the circulatory system. An increase in blood volume raises blood pressure.

The Uric Acid Controversy

More than 100 studies demonstrate that people with high uric acid are at increased risk for developing and dying from heart disease, as well as other arterial diseases. So why don't doctors check your uric acid when they measure cholesterol and other blood factors? Because despite strong evidence indicting elevated uric acid as a serious health threat, no major medical association currently recommends routine screening for levels of this rogue molecule. That includes the American Heart Association, the American Diabetes Association, and the National Kidney Foundation, among other leading medical groups. None of these organizations considers uric acid to be an important risk factor for obesity, heart disease, diabetes, or any other major disease. Why?

There are several reasons that the present-day medical establishment has not embraced uric acid screening as a way to identify patients at heightened risk for heart disease and other conditions. Here are the three main arguments against measuring uric acid, with my response to each.

The chicken-or-egg argument

It is undeniable that many people with high uric acid levels are overweight and have other serious metabolic problems. But which comes first? Skeptics point out that in some cases, uric acid levels rise *after* a person has developed certain conditions of metabolic syndrome. For example, the prediabetic condition called hyperinsulinemia, or elevated insulin levels, can increase uric acid. Likewise, diminished blood flow to the kidneys, which occurs in people who develop hypertension, reduces the amount of uric acid that's excreted in urine. In turn, blood levels of uric acid rise. These two phenomena suggest that high uric acid is a by-product of metabolic syndrome—not the cause.

On the other hand: Studies have also shown that a rise in uric acid often occurs *before* people gain weight or develop high blood pressure or diabetes. In these cases, high uric acid can't be a by-product of these conditions, because it occurred first.

The "uric acid is good" argument

Some scientists think that uric acid is, at worst, harmless. Others say it may even be beneficial. Surprisingly, uric acid can act as an antioxidant—that is, it can neutralize the effects of destructive molecules called free radicals. Your body generates free radicals during normal metabolism; exposure to environmental toxins—such as tobacco smoke or pollution—causes levels to rise, too. Free radicals are responsible for the cell damage known as oxidation, which raises the risk for cardiovascular disease, cancer, and other conditions. Some research suggests that uric acid can reverse oxidative damage. If this is true, then a rise in uric acid might actually be a good thing—your body's way of combating disease.

On the other hand: In low concentrations, uric acid may indeed promote health, perhaps by functioning as an antioxidant. But we know that laboratory animals given fructose show a rise in uric acid, which causes them to gain weight and develop high blood pressure, insulin resistance, and other conditions of metabolic syndrome. Strong scientific evidence suggests that the same thing happens to humans who elevate their uric acid by eating a diet that's too high in fructose or purines.

The independent risk factor argument

Some researchers have argued that uric acid cannot be considered a cause of cardiovascular disease because it does not act directly, through a unique mechanism. They point out that high uric acid usually accompanies some other condition that raises the risk for heart attack, such as hypertension or kidney disease. If uric acid does not *independently* cause cardiovascular disease, they ask, why bother measuring it?

One influential argument against using uric acid to screen for heart disease came from the famous Framingham Heart Study, which has been evaluating the cardiovascular health of a group of people from a city outside Boston since 1948. A team of scientists analyzed data from the Framingham study using a statistical technique that isolated the effects of elevated uric acid from other potential risk factors for heart disease. They determined that high uric acid did not appear to cause heart attacks.

The group published their findings in the *Annals of Internal Medicine* in 1999. Their paper had a major influence on physicians' perceptions about the value of screening for uric acid, which is not surprising. After all, during its history, the Framingham study has made major contributions to the prevention of heart attacks, such as linking cigarette smoking and elevated cholesterol to cardiovascular disease. If scientists involved in this important study say that measuring uric acid levels serves no purpose, most doctors will be inclined to believe them.

On the other hand: Although some studies have failed to show that uric acid is an independent risk factor for heart disease, others have reached the opposite conclusion. Besides, let's assume for a moment that uric acid does not cause heart disease directly. This does not mean that it can't raise your risk *indirectly.* After all, strong evidence tells us that uric acid makes you gain weight and develop hypertension— both of which raise the risk for heart attack. The authors of the influential *Annals of Internal Medicine* paper did not consider this possibility.

Beyond Uric Acid

A high-fructose diet makes you gain weight and creates metabolic chaos—but it does not act solely by raising uric acid. Indeed, we have discovered that fructose performs much of its damage through other pathways. In the next chapter, I'll describe how fructose exploits your sensitive palate, tricks your hormones, slows down your metabolism, and—perhaps most important—revs up enzymes that make your fat cells fatter and your overall health suffer.

CHAPTER 6

SUGAR SHOCK

How Fructose Makes You Fat

It's not your fault.

That's my message to anyone who has ever struggled to lose weight, or fought even harder to keep it from returning—and failed. Losing weight can be a great challenge. And surveys consistently show that most people who manage to shed pounds eventually regain at least some of the weight, if not all.

Unfortunately, many people assume that weight problems and the failure of weight-loss diets are due to a lack of self-control. Social commentators insist that the unprecedented rise in obesity rates that has occurred in the United States over the past generation is not so much a medical crisis as an epidemic of overindulgence and moral weakness.

This perspective is especially strong overseas. I often travel abroad, both to give lectures and for pleasure. In recent years, I have visited Brazil, Egypt, Japan, New Zealand, Singapore, Spain, and Turkey. Inevitably, I find that people in foreign countries often look upon the United States as the land of lost willpower, a nation of people with no backbone or inner fortitude. They think that millions of Americans are overweight because our self-restraint wilts when we're faced with the huge portions of food our restaurants serve. They believe that obesity is a character issue, and they find ours lacking.

Nonsense. We are not by nature a population of undisciplined gluttons. There is nothing wrong with our national resolve. Americans are gaining weight at the current unhealthy and dangerous rate because we find ourselves living in an environment that is changing in important ways—some obvious, some less so.

For starters, the modern world makes gaining weight altogether too easy. Evolution gave us bodies programmed to seek and stockpile calories in fat tissue as a backup energy source in case of famine. Yet the famine never comes. Instead, we live in a land of plenty, where a Burger King Double Whopper with Cheese (1,150 calories) or large Dairy Queen Oreo Blizzard (more than 1,010 calories) isn't more than a short drive away for most Americans.

Indeed, unlike our prehistoric ancestors, we are literally surrounded by food. There are nearly a million restaurants in the United States. The typical supermarket sells 50,000 food products, with some 20,000 new products introduced each year.

Then again, it's not as though we walk, much less jog, to the nearest restaurant or grocery. Lack of exercise and the proliferation of laborsaving devices have resulted in an overall drop in physical activity among Americans, ensuring that many of the calories we store so efficiently in our fat tissue remain there.

But while the easy availability of high-calorie foods and our relatively sedentary lifestyles have without question contributed to the rising tide of obesity in the United States, I believe there is more to the story. Another element has entered the picture and driven the sudden surge in weight gain in this country over the past generation. The stealth factor is fructose and its unique effect on human metabolism.

Persuasive scientific evidence shows that fructose "tricks" the body into gaining weight and keeping the pounds in place. I believe that the typical American diet makes the body ultrasensitive to sugar, high-fructose corn syrup (HFCS), and other sources of fructose. Eventually, eating even small amounts of fructose triggers a metabolic response that creates persistent hunger, overeating, and fat accumulation. This simple sugar exerts its powerful influence on your weight in a number of ways.

- Fructose increases palatability—that is, it makes food tasty and appetizing—which coaxes you into eating more calories than your body needs.

- Unlike other forms of sugar, fructose does not trigger the release of important hormone signals to areas of the brain that control appetite. In other words, even large servings of fructose-rich foods leave you hungry.

- Over a long period, eating too much fructose may block your brain from responding to hormones that control appetite—*even when you eat foods that don't contain fructose.* In other words, a high-fructose diet can cause your brain to become resistant to the normal, healthy signals that tell you to stop eating. As a result, you may tend to eat too much of all kinds of foods, including fat and protein.

- Fructose damages healthy fat cells, making them sickly and causing them to fill up with excessive amounts of fat.

- Eating fructose causes levels of critical enzymes to rise and become more active, which exaggerates the effects of even small amounts of sugar in the diet.

- Some evidence suggests that eating foods with fructose may cause greater weight gain than other types of foods, even when you consume the same number of calories. Fructose may produce this unwelcome effect by either altering how efficiently your body burns calories or increasing how rapidly your body absorbs certain foods (specifically glucose).

Of course, eating too much of any food will make you gain weight. That's particularly true if you consume a lot of high-fat foods; after all, fat provides more than twice as many calories per gram (9 calories) as carbohydrates and protein (4 calories). Studies confirm what might seem like an obvious equation: If you eat a high-fat diet, you will indeed become overweight or obese. Over time, however, as your cells fill up with fat, you will likely develop more serious complications, such as insulin resistance and high blood pressure, which can raise your risk for diabetes and heart disease.

A high-fructose diet actually turns around this process, causing you to gain weight through a different pathway—though the results are the same as for a high-fat diet. When you eat too much fructose, your fat cells become sick and

OBESITY, DEFINED

The Centers for Disease Control and Prevention defines obesity as having a body mass index, or BMI, of 30 or higher. A person is overweight if his or her BMI falls between 25 and 29.

HEIGHT	WEIGHT (LB)													
5'0"	97	102	107	112	118	123	128	133	138	143	148	153	158	163
5'1"	100	106	111	116	122	127	132	137	143	148	153	158	164	169
5'2"	104	109	115	120	126	131	136	142	147	153	158	164	169	175
5'3"	107	113	118	124	130	135	141	146	152	158	163	169	175	180
5'4"	110	116	122	128	134	140	145	151	157	163	169	174	180	186
5'5"	114	120	126	132	138	144	150	156	162	168	174	180	186	192
5'6"	118	124	130	136	142	148	155	161	167	173	179	186	192	198
5'7"	121	127	134	140	146	153	159	166	172	178	185	191	198	204
5'8"	125	131	138	144	151	158	164	171	177	184	190	197	203	210
5'9"	128	135	142	149	155	162	169	176	182	189	196	203	209	216
5'10"	132	139	146	153	160	167	174	181	188	195	202	209	216	222
5'11"	136	143	150	157	165	172	179	186	193	200	208	215	222	229
6'0"	140	147	154	162	169	177	184	191	199	206	213	221	228	235
6'1"	144	151	159	166	174	182	189	197	204	212	219	227	235	242
6'2"	148	155	163	171	179	186	194	202	210	218	225	233	241	249
BMI	19	20	21	22	23	24	25	26	27	28	29	30	31	32

unhealthy *first*, well before you begin to gain weight. In fact, even if you are normal in size now, overloading your body with fructose may be inducing changes in your fat cells that could eventually cause you to gain a lot of weight. If you are already overweight, then consuming even moderate amounts of sugar, HFCS, and other sources of fructose may be the reason you can't slim down.

Let's take a closer look at the unique properties of fructose to better understand why sweet foods expand your waistline.

The Curse of Good Taste: Fructose and Palatability

Here are the two least-controversial statements you will read in this entire book: Fructose makes food taste good, and once you start eating a tasty food, stopping can be difficult. As a result, it's easy to overindulge when you eat sweets.

But isn't this true of other foods, too? After all, isn't there some truth to that old advertising jingle—the one that dares you to eat just one potato chip? And doesn't devouring one slice of pepperoni pizza beckon you to go back for more?

To be sure, fat and saltiness also make food highly palatable, which is the scientific way of describing dishes we find mouthwatering and irresistible. But scientists who study food preferences say that humans show a great range in their desire to eat dishes that are high in fat or salt. That is, people in some cultures don't find potato chips, pizza, or other salty or fatty foods terribly mouthwatering or irresistible. In contrast, a taste for sweetness appears to be universal. If you visit the most exotic, far-flung location on the planet and offer a chocolate bar to the first person you meet, you will undoubtedly make a new friend.

Research also strongly suggests that a love of sweetness is programmed into the brains of all mammals, probably so that infants will instinctively nurse on mother's milk (which has a slightly sweet taste because it contains lactose, or milk sugar). In prehistoric times, when humans needed to hunt and forage for their meals, palatability and nutritional value were closely linked. That is, the best-tasting foods, such as sweet, ripe fructose-rich fruit, were the healthiest foods, too. On the other hand, humans and other mammals appear to be prewired to avoid sourness, probably to keep from eating spoiled fruit, and bitterness, to protect against eating toxic plants. Of course, we've overcome our innate resistance to sour and bitter foods. But is it any wonder that biting into a lemon makes us wince?

The natural human preference for sweetness has been demonstrated in many experiments. For example, studies show that newborns suckle more enthusiastically when given water sweetened with sucrose (which is half fructose) than when given water flavored with glucose. Likewise, infants consume more formula if it is sweetened with sugar than if it tastes bland.

There is little doubt that sweetness affects our emotions. Studies have shown, for instance, that crying newborns calm down when given a sweetened liquid but continue to wail when fed an unflavored beverage. The yearning for sweet foods seems to intensify as we age. In *The Botany of Desire: A Plant's-Eye View of the World,* author Michael Pollan describes the first time his son tasted sugar, in the form of icing on the cake at his first birthday party.

[H]e was beside himself with the pleasure of it, no longer here with me in space and time in quite the same way he had been just a moment before. Between bites, Isaac gazed up at me in amazement (he was on my lap, and I was delivering the ambrosial forkfuls to his gaping mouth) as if to exclaim, "Your world contains this? From this day forward, I shall dedicate my life to it." (Which he basically has done.) And I remember thinking, this is no minor desire, and then wondered: Could it be that sweetness is the prototype of *all* desire?

Unfortunately, there's a downside to this sweet ecstasy. Consuming highly palatable food such as fructose appears to cause many of the same behaviors and neurochemical changes in the brain that occur in the brains of people who use addictive drugs. For example, in a study from researchers at Princeton University, laboratory rats that had grown accustomed to consuming sugar-laced water and chow became anxious and developed withdrawal-like symptoms—such as chattering teeth and tremors—when deprived of sweets for an extended period. When these foods were returned to the rats' diets, they ate and drank nonstop, greedily filling themselves.

The Princeton group also found that during these sugar binges, the rats produced high levels of the neurotransmitter dopamine in a region of the brain believed to govern pleasure—the same thing that happens in the brains of people who use amphetamines and cocaine. In addition, sugar bingeing seems to produce brain changes similar to those caused by opiate drugs, such as heroin and morphine. In studies using MRI and positron emission tomography scans, humans experienced the same sort of alterations in brain function after consuming sugar that occur in drug addicts.

Clearly, fructose's high palatability has its benefits, because it makes nutritious foods such as fruit and (to a lesser extent) vegetables more appealing to eat. Yet fructose makes jelly beans, root beer, and chocolate chip cookies hard to resist, too. The craving for sweet foods not only can make you consume too many calories and gain weight, it also can flood your body with fructose, causing a variety of unhealthy metabolic changes that compromise your ability to maintain a healthy weight.

But great taste isn't the only reason we tend to eat too much fructose. This simple sugar also foils the efforts of your body's appetite-control system, as you will see next.

Fructose and Appetite: The Hormone Connection

Unlike other animals, humans have created rituals surrounding the act of eating. If you're like most people, you probably consume three meals per day, set apart by intervals of several hours, in the morning, afternoon, and early evening, with occasional snacks in between. At least a few times a year, you may eat special dinners to celebrate holidays, such as Thanksgiving and Passover. Food also plays a central role in many of our most cherished customs, from weddings to trick-or-treating to watching the Super Bowl.

Apart from the social importance of food and dining, however, we eat for one obvious reason: because we're hungry. Unfortunately, fructose fails us on this basic level, because it does a poor job of satisfying hunger. For some reason, your body's appetite-control system ignores fructose, which makes it a kind of phantom food ingredient. As a result, when you eat a high-fructose food, your appetite does not become satisfied, so you may keep eating. Perhaps worse, emerging research from studies conducted by my group and other investigators indicate that a high-fructose diet can actually interfere with important signaling systems in the brain that control your appetite for *all* foods.

Before I explain why fructose's stealthy metabolic status does little to quiet a growling stomach, let's take a look at how your body regulates the amount of food you eat. Scientists used to think that weight gain was simple to explain: Eat too much food, and you get fat. Though we still believe that consuming more calories than you burn off through physical activity leads to weight gain, it has become clear that the amount of food you eat is governed by a complex biological system that involves several key hormones. Researchers have discovered that different foods influence the behavior of these hormones in unique ways. In other words, what foods you choose may influence how much you eat.

When you eat a meal containing carbohydrates, glucose is absorbed from the gastrointestinal tract and enters the bloodstream. Cells use glucose to create energy. As blood glucose levels rise, the pancreas produces insulin. This important hormone ushers glucose into cells, which in turn lowers blood glucose levels.

Insulin is a busy hormone, with a variety of important roles in the body. One of its other tasks is to trigger the release of a hormone called leptin from fat cells. Named for *leptos*, the Greek word for thin, leptin rises in proportion to the amount of fat stored by your body. It acts directly on the brain cells that are believed to control satiety, or the pleasant sensation of fullness you feel after a meal. At the same time, insulin turns down production of ghrelin, a hormone in the stomach that appears to promote hunger. Together, levels of these hormones deliver a signal to the brain: Your appetite has been satisfied, so stop eating.

Both glucose and fructose are simple sugars, but they differ in many significant ways. Here's an important one: Fructose does not trigger the pancreas to release large amounts of insulin into the blood. This distinction may seem appealing to people with diabetes, whose bodies have difficulty processing glucose. But this unique characteristic also poses a problem. Because fructose doesn't cause a steep rise in insulin, it causes only modest, if any, changes in leptin and ghrelin. The result? Food and beverages that are high in fructose provide plenty of calories, but they do a poor job of satisfying your appetite. Instead, they leave you feeling hungry, which may lead you to overeat.

We know that fructose has little or no effect on appetite hormones—and, more important, on your appetite—thanks to a landmark study by nutritionist Peter J. Havel, PhD, of the University of California at Davis. Dr. Havel and several colleagues recruited a dozen women to participate in their study. Each of the women reported to a laboratory twice, a month apart, for two nights at a time. On the first day of each session, the subjects consumed a limited amount of food. On the next day, the researchers encouraged the women to eat as much as they wished from a selection of different foods. But during one visit, the study participants drank beverages sweetened with glucose on the first day. During the other session, they washed down their meals with fructose-sweetened drinks on the first day.

The purpose of Dr. Havel's study was to examine how fructose and glucose affected the women's hunger levels, appetite hormones, and food choices. The team measured the women's hunger by asking questions such as "How full is your stomach right now?" and "How much food could you eat right now?" They also took blood samples at various times throughout the study. On the all-you-can-eat day, they measured how much and what types of foods the women consumed.

The results: Blood tests showed that the women's leptin levels were 35 percent lower when they drank fructose-sweetened beverages than when they drank glucose beverages. Likewise, the fructose drinks had little effect on ghrelin levels. What's more, the women reported feeling hungrier on the day they drank the fructose beverages. Not surprisingly, they ate larger amounts of high-fat foods the day after drinking the fructose beverages, suggesting that their bodies craved calories. (Remember, fat has twice as many calories as protein and carbohydrates.)

As part of Dr. Havel's study, the women filled out questionnaires describing their dietary habits. Women whom the scientists determined to be "restrained eaters" were most affected by drinking the high-fructose beverages; that is, they felt hungrier and ate more the next day than women identified as "unrestrained eaters." Psychologists use the phrase "restrained eater" to describe chronic dieters who make an effort to limit the amount of food they eat, but who frequently overeat if they feel stressed out or become distracted. Unrestrained eaters simply stop eating when they feel satisfied and do not attempt to count calories or limit food intake. This suggests that consuming fructose-rich foods and beverages may be an especially bad idea if you're actively trying to lose weight, because they seem to encourage overeating.

The study's bottom line: Because leptin and ghrelin ap-

pear to ignore fructose, your body still feels hungry after
you have consumed large amounts of this simple sugar. As
a result, you keep eating, even though your energy demands
have been met and your fuel tank is full. Obviously, this
means you are taking in excess calories, which your body
will store in the form of fat.

Halting the Hunger-Control Hormones: Leptin Resistance

In addition to eluding the attention of leptin, fructose seems
to block this appetite hormone from doing its job, which
makes maintaining a healthy weight even harder. A problem known as leptin resistance occurs when the hormone is
unable to deliver its "stop eating" message to the brain. As a
result, a person with leptin resistance may consume more
food than he or she needs to satisfy appetite, which can
cause weight gain. Studies indicate that obese people often
show evidence of leptin resistance.

High doses of fructose cause leptin resistance. This
phenomenon was demonstrated in a 2008 study led by two
of my former colleagues at the University of Florida, Alex-
andra Shapiro, PhD, and Philip Scarpace, PhD. My group
collaborated with Drs. Shapiro and Scarpace on this research. We fed laboratory rats a high-fructose diet for 6
months. Next, we injected the rats with leptin. The hormone had little effect on the rats' appetite. They kept right
on eating, indicating that they had become leptin resistant.

What happened during the next stage of the study tells
us a great deal about the far-reaching effects of a high-
fructose diet. We switched the leptin-resistant rats to a high-
fat, Western-style diet. We also fed the same diet to a group
of similar rats that were not leptin resistant. The results were

striking: The rats with fructose-induced leptin resistance ate more and gained much more weight, faster, than the control rats.

So now we know of two ways fructose can sabotage your appetite hormones. First, as I explained earlier, leptin levels do not rise sharply when you consume high-fructose foods. As a result, fructose-rich meals do a poor job of satisfying appetite. Your fat cells *do* produce leptin when you consume other foods, of course. That brings me to the second problem: Our study and other research offer evidence that chronic consumption of high-fructose foods can cause lep-

---

CELLULITE AND FRUCTOSE

Could cutting back on fructose help relieve a familiar cosmetic problem? Cellulite is a condition that creates a dimpled or "cottage cheese" appearance in the skin, usually on the hips, thighs, or buttocks. Cellulite is most common in females, though it doesn't appear until after puberty. Cellulite usually affects males only if they develop a condition that lowers their testosterone, such as Klinefelter's syndrome (characterized by the presence of an extra X chromosome). No one knows for sure what causes cellulite, though these patterns suggest that hormones play a role. Other factors are probably involved as well.

Research suggests that the layer of fat underlying skin with cellulite often develops many of the same metabolic problems that have been linked to a high-fructose diet. For example, studies show that in people with cellulite, fat cells in the subcutaneous layer of skin can be highly inflamed. We know from our research that exposing fat cells to fructose or uric acid can cause the cells to become inflamed and develop oxidative stress. Some research has linked cellulite to diets high in carbohydrates. It's possible that one carbohydrate in particular, fructose, could be the culprit.

We still have much to learn about the link between cellulite and fructose. However, the many so-called cellulite cures on the market are either unproven or ineffective. We know that a low-fructose diet will help you lose weight and improve overall health. Research may eventually show that it also blocks the inflammation in fat cells that's associated with cellulite.

tin resistance, which prevents the hormone from turning off appetite, no matter what kinds of foods you eat.

How does fructose block leptin? We don't know, but it may be that fructose affects the blood-brain barrier. This layer of tightly packed blood vessels regulates which substances pass into the brain. As I explained in Chapter 5, high levels of uric acid generated when you eat fructose shut down production of nitric oxide in blood vessels, which causes them to constrict. It's possible that this narrowing of vessels in the blood-brain barrier keeps leptin from reaching its destination. Studies suggest that high levels of triglycerides may also induce leptin resistance at the blood-brain barrier, too. Finally, it may be that fructose affects how the brain cells respond to leptin.

Cell Shock:
Fructose and Stress inside the Cell

As I mentioned earlier, some people eat too much—especially high-fat comfort foods—when they feel stressed out. In a sense, your fat cells react the same way when you consume fructose. The act of processing this simple sugar is very taxing for cells, leaving them exhausted and sick. When cells are sapped of energy, they can't function properly. To prevent future fructose-induced power outages, they produce a dense source of energy: fat. This is why, over time, a high-fructose diet causes fat tissue to get bigger and bulkier.

This is my theory about how the act of metabolizing fructose produces flab and ruins diets. While we can't say for certain why cells fill up with fat in response to a "hit" of fructose, both our research and the work of other groups support the idea that they do it as a means of self-preservation. Unfortunately, as fat cells protect themselves from the

WHAT IS INFLAMMATION?

When you consume a large amount of fructose, the tissues in your body become inflamed. You don't develop immediate and obvious symptoms the way you do during a bout of acute inflammation, such as the red, prickly skin that is characteristic of dermatitis or the aches and pains that accompany a sinus infection. Instead, fructose triggers low-grade systemic inflammation, which can produce silent but devastating damage throughout your body.

Inflammation isn't all bad, of course. You couldn't survive without it, because it is an essential component of your body's defense network. Any time you are injured or an unwelcome intruder such as a germ or toxin finds its way into your body, your immune system swings into action, producing a variety of chemicals that control damage and speed up healing. Histamines, for example, increase blood flow to the site of injury or infection. White blood cells, meanwhile, destroy bacteria and other microorganisms while helping to repair injured cells.

But glitches can develop in the immune system, causing the body to attack itself. The result is an autoimmune disorder, in which inflammatory chemicals destroy healthy tissue, as is the case in rheumatoid arthritis (which affects the joints) or lupus erythematosus (the connective tissue).

In recent years, it has become clear that chronic, low-grade inflammation is a stealth factor in other, more common diseases. For example, we now know atherosclerosis to be an inflammatory disease. Groundbreaking research has demonstrated that silent, persistent inflammation contributes to the narrowing of arteries that leads to heart attack and stroke. Blood tests reveal that people who have high blood pressure and other features of metabolic syndrome, as well

withering effects of fructose, your waistline and overall health may suffer.

Much of what we know about fructose's role in weight gain springs from our evolving understanding of body fat. Until about 20 years ago, most scientists believed that fat tissue was little more than storage space. The theory was simple: When you eat more calories than you burn off through physical activity, your body tucks away the excess energy in fat cells, like filling the shelves of a pantry with food for another day. In the old way of thinking, fat just sat there, static and inactive.

We have since learned that fat tissue is not simply a doras kidney disease, tend to have low-grade inflammation, too. What's more, strong evidence suggests that inflammation is an underlying cause of several types of cancer.

Yet a daunting question remains unanswered: What causes systemic inflammation? There is probably no single answer, but fructose appears to play a role.

According to research from our laboratory, the amount of fructose that you might ingest from a fast-food meal can cause the cells in blood vessels to become inflamed, which can trigger heart attacks. We have identified the same phenomenon in kidney cells, liver cells, and fat cells exposed to fructose.

Fructose appears to set the stage for inflammation via several mechanisms. We know that cells exposed to fructose become temporarily depleted of energy, which can cause them to become inflamed. We also know that fructose triggers the endothelial cells lining the inner walls of arteries to produce factors that attract white blood cells, contributing to inflammation. What's more, fructose stimulates the production of uric acid. Studies show that uric acid can directly induce inflammation inside the arteries.

Laboratory studies reveal that even small amounts of fructose can cause changes in blood vessels and fat tissue that raise levels of inflammation. Once again, it's a low-grade, symptomless form of inflammation, so drinking a soda or a tall glass of fruit juice will not leave you feeling sore or turn your skin red, as an acute inflammatory condition might. Nonetheless, chronic inflammation is a serious problem with far-reaching consequences for your health.

mant, inert storage compartment for excess calories. In fact, fat is a highly active, thriving organ that is teeming with hormones, enzymes, and other proteins that help to control normal energy metabolism. Ideally, the chemicals generated by fat tissue work to keep your body weight in balance. In other words, your fat tissue actually helps to prevent you from becoming . . . well . . . fat.

Eating a fructose-rich food disrupts this healthy balance by causing destructive changes to fat cells. The trouble begins not long after you guzzle a bottle of cola, finish off a sugary dessert, savor a juicy orange, or consume any other source of fructose. That's because your body processes fructose very quickly. As soon as it enters your cells, enzymes set upon fructose and immediately break it down in order to create energy. In the process, fructose causes cells to rapidly burn up energy-producing molecules called adenosine triphosphate, or ATP.

Have you ever felt a burst of energy after eating a large candy bar or swigging down a soda? That's because your cells are producing heat as they rapidly burn up ATP. Think of ATP as "currency," because it determines how much power a cell can generate.

With this analogy in mind, fructose is an "expensive" food, because cells must spend a great deal of ATP to metabolize it. In one study, doctors gave surgery patients 50 grams of fructose by intravenous infusion, which is slightly less than the typical American consumes in a day. Liver biopsies showed that the fructose lowered ATP levels by about half. Eating a high-fructose meal, then, could drain much of your cells' energy bank account, quickly. When cells become depleted of ATP, your energy level slumps, and you develop that familiar postsugar depression.

Starved of energy, cells go into a state of shock. We have exposed human cells to fructose in laboratory studies, and the effect is stunning—literally. Activity in the cells shuts down, as though they had lost their blood supply. In fact, cells begin to act as though they were suffering ischemia, a loss of blood flow that leads to cell death and causes most heart attacks and strokes. Fructose does not cut off blood supply, however. Instead, it shocks cells from the inside, leaving them temporarily unable to function.

And that's only the beginning of the trouble. As you'll recall from the previous chapter, as cells burn up ATP, they generate uric acid, with all of its ill effects. What's more, cells depleted of ATP become inflamed. Oxidative stress also occurs as molecules called free radicals are generated and interact with uric acid and other cell components, which further damages cells. Our research shows that the amount of fructose in a large soft drink can trigger all of these damaging changes in a variety of cell types, including fat cells, liver cells, and the cells that line blood vessels.

A cell stunned by fructose is a cell in crisis. The sense of

WHAT IS OXIDATIVE STRESS?

Eating a high-fructose diet is one of many ways to increase oxidative stress, a destructive phenomenon linked to many diseases. Every moment, with every breath, your body produces toxic chemicals called free radicals, which damage healthy tissue through a process called oxidation. Although oxygen is necessary to produce life-sustaining energy, a small percentage of the oxygen you inhale ends up generating free radicals. Exposure to environmental toxins such as air pollution, cigarette smoke, and radiation contributes to oxidative stress, too.

Free radicals are unstable particles that are missing electrons. They try to restore lost electrons by stealing a pair from any tissue in their path. Left unchecked, free radicals can oxidize cholesterol, which causes this waxy substance to clog arteries. Oxidation also seems to promote high blood pressure. Free radicals may injure cell membranes and DNA, which is why many scientists believe that oxidative stress plays a role in cancer and aging itself.

Ideally, our bodies keep oxidation to a minimum by staying well stocked with defenders called antioxidants, which defuse free radicals. Your body manufactures some antioxidant compounds and enzymes, but others must come from a healthy diet. Some vitamins—beta-carotene, vitamin C, and vitamin E—act as antioxidants, as do a few minerals, such as selenium. Certain plant chemicals, known as phytochemicals, also have antioxidant powers. Two you may have heard of are lycopene (found in tomatoes, watermelon, and other foods) and resveratrol (in red wine and peanuts).

Unfortunately, this antioxidant defense system can become overwhelmed by high levels of free-radical activity. This unhealthy imbalance is known as oxidative stress. Eating a high-fructose diet contributes to this problem. As a cell metabolizes fructose and uses up its ATP, the cell's uric acid levels rise. Free radicals are produced and interact with uric acid, leading to the creation of even more radicals and producing high levels of oxidative stress.

panic is greatest in your fat tissue and certain other organs, which—as you will learn in the next section—are most sensitive to fructose. How do they respond? By filling up with fat, as well as glycogen, the storage form of glucose. Although we can only speculate why this happens, it may be a cell's way of protecting itself against the starvation brought on when fructose drains its ATP. From a fat cell's perspective, storing large amounts of fat may allow it to weather the storm the next time fructose strikes.

Unfortunately, this is an unhealthy form of protection. Obviously, as fat cells get fatter, so do you. What's more, as cells fill up with fat, they resist the effects of insulin. This means they will have difficulty using glucose, the body's preferred energy source. Ironically, even though fructose doesn't prompt your body to produce a large amount of insulin following a meal, your insulin level may eventually rise if you eat a high-fructose diet for an extended period. That's because chronic fructose consumption induces insulin resistance. In response, the pancreas pours more insulin into the blood, causing levels of the hormone to rise. Insulin resistance is a serious problem, because it serves as a prelude to type 2 diabetes, hypertension, and heart disease.

It's worth noting here that the glucose in starchy foods may cause blood glucose levels to rise, which stimulates the pancreas to produce insulin. But this is normal and healthy. Dietary glucose does *not* cause insulin resistance; fructose does.

Fructose and Metabolism

Eating too much fructose may cause your body to burn calories less efficiently. Over time, this could cause you to gain weight. Here's why: Some research suggests that fructose lowers your body's basal metabolic rate, or BMR, which is the number of calories you use at rest.

You may not realize it, but you burn calories all day long, whether you're huffing and puffing on a treadmill or dozing in a hammock. This is because the many physiological processes that keep your organs running and tissue nourished require energy, even when you sleep.

BMR is an important factor in weight management. As a rule, your BMR gradually declines as you get older, which is one reason why many people who never needed to worry about their weight suddenly find themselves fighting flab as they enter middle age and beyond.

I believe that eating a high-fructose diet may have a similar effect. Cells metabolize fructose very quickly. In the process, they lose ATP, the molecules that serve as the main power source for metabolism. Unfortunately, as your ATP levels sink, so does your metabolic rate. This means that a high-fructose diet could depress your metabolic rate.

If true, this would help explain studies like the one I mentioned in Chapter 3, in which children who drank lots of fructose-rich fruit juice were more likely to be obese than kids who consumed less fructose but the same number of calories. Your weight is a reflection not only of the calories you eat but also of the calories you burn, so if your metabolic rate drops, weight gain will result. Indeed, the same phenomenon has been shown in laboratory studies: Mice fed fructose-rich diets gain more weight than mice that eat the same amount of fructose-free food.

There is a second possible explanation for why you gain more weight when you consume fructose than when you take in an equal amount of calories from other foods. Research has shown that fructose enhances the absorption of glucose. This suggests that the fructose in sugar and HFCS may cause you to absorb more glucose than you would when eating a meal of an equal amount of starch, which breaks down to glucose.

We need to study this question more closely. If, indeed, fructose lowers your BMR, you will be less likely to burn off the calories from sugar and other sources of fructose through normal daily metabolism. Unless you start exercising more or eating less, weight gain is inevitable.

Priming Your Fat Cells: Fructose and Enzymes

Much of the blame for the growing epidemic of obesity in the United States and around the world has been traced to the popularity of cheap burgers, tacos, and other fast foods. In a way, fructose is the ultimate "fast" food, because your body processes it so rapidly. Unfortunately, if you are flooding your system with fructose by eating too many sugary foods, the enzymes required to break it down may respond by becoming overactive. This could cause your body to set in motion the metabolic changes that cause weight gain every time you consume fructose, even just a small amount.

Enzymes are the body's catalysts. These various proteins initiate an unfathomable number of biological reactions that are necessary for the healthy functioning of every organ system. One enzyme in particular, called fructokinase, helps to convert fructose into energy. Fructokinase—which I'll simply call fructose enzymes—is present in tissue cells throughout the body, with the highest concentrations in certain organs, including the liver, intestines, and kidneys. High levels of fructose enzymes are also present in fat cells.

Fructose enzymes may turn fructose into energy, but they do so at a high price. As I explained earlier, cells generate a rogue's gallery of destructive compounds as they metabolize fructose. In particular, we know that burning fructose generates uric acid, which has been linked to weight gain, among other metabolic problems. Unfortunately, if you eat large amounts of foods containing fructose every day, your body responds by manufacturing a huge volume of fructose enzymes. This makes your cells overly sensitive, causing them to generate large amounts of uric acid every time you consume sugar. It's as though your body's machinery for manufacturing uric acid and other damaging compounds got stuck in high gear.

Similarly, your intestines absorb fructose through specific transport proteins. One of the main transport proteins, called Glut-5, also increases in number if you consume a high-fructose diet over a long period. As your Glut-5 levels increase, your body absorbs more fructose any time you consume foods or beverages that contain the sugar.

A small study published in the British medical journal *Lancet* illustrates how the body can become ultrasensitive to fructose. Researchers gave a fructose beverage to volunteers who had adopted a low-fructose diet, then measured their uric acid levels. Blood tests showed that uric acid rose modestly. When the researchers repeated this test on volunteers who had been eating a high-fructose diet, the results were quite different: The same fructose drink caused a much greater rise in uric acid levels. Apparently, avoiding fructose in the diet kept fructose enzymes under control,

ESSENTIAL FRUCTOSURIA: BETTER THAN BENIGN?

What if you didn't have fructose enzymes? This is the case for the roughly 120,000 people in the United States with a condition called essential fructosuria. Because they lack fructokinase, people who have this rare inherited disorder can consume large amounts of fructose without producing uric acid. Nor are they at risk for "cell shock," because eating fructose does not cause their cells to burn up energy stores. People with essential fructosuria lose between 10 and 20 percent of the fructose they consume in their urine, but this is harmless.

Essential fructosuria is a benign condition; most people who have it are perfectly healthy. In fact, one Swiss researcher is tracking a large extended family in which several members have essential fructosuria—and none of them is overweight.

which in turn kept uric acid levels low. On the other hand, eating a high-fructose diet turned up the volume on fructose enzymes, making them overreact and generating excessive amounts of uric acid.

As I explained in the previous chapter, high uric acid levels are closely linked to obesity, which is why my colleagues and I are studying fructokinase and other related enzymes. Learning more about fructose enzymes may help to explain why some people become fat and others don't. It could be, for instance, that certain people have naturally elevated fructose enzymes. It is possible that populations such as the Pima Indians of New Mexico—with their shockingly high rates of obesity and diabetes—have a genetic defect that causes them to produce high levels of fructose enzymes and therefore makes them unusually vulnerable to sugar, HFCS, and other sweeteners. My colleagues and I are exploring how genetics influences the behavior of fructokinase and other enzymes.

It's possible that learning how to control and regulate

fructokinase could have a profound effect on the epidemic of obesity and metabolic syndrome gripping the United States and many parts of the world. One day, we may be able to develop drugs that are capable of blocking fructose enzymes, which would allow us to prevent them from raising uric acid and producing other damaging effects.

For now, however, there is a simple way to lower the volume and reduce the activity of fructose enzymes on your own—by choosing the right foods. I'll explain how to do just that in Chapter 11.

CHAPTER 7

THE (OTHER) TROUBLE WITH FRUCTOSE

More Ways That the Low-Fructose Diet Will Improve Your Health

The science is clear and powerful: Cutting back on fructose will help maintain a healthy weight and control the various conditions of metabolic syndrome, such as high blood pressure and elevated blood glucose—in turn, lowering your risk for heart disease, diabetes, and other health concerns. But these may not be the only perks of switching to a low-fructose diet.

Some of the collateral health benefits of reducing your fructose consumption will likely seem obvious. Refined sugar is half fructose, of course, and as every schoolchild knows, eating sugary foods promotes tooth decay—especially if you don't brush and floss regularly. (All the same, I would encourage you to read the section about fructose and your teeth to learn why even some sugar-free products can damage your dentition.)

On the other hand, much of what you read in this chapter may come as a surprise. For instance, if you are plagued by mysterious digestive problems even though you have sworn off spicy foods, you may find that your stomach discomfort diminishes or disappears when you stop overloading your system with fructose.

Other possible benefits of lowering your fructose intake are less immediate and evident, though they could have an even greater payoff. Some research implicates sugar, and fructose in particular, as a contributing factor in several common forms of cancer, for example. What's more, cutting-edge science shows that fructose fuels the formation of molecules that may help to regulate the aging process. We could eventually learn that eating and drinking too much fructose makes you grow old before your time.

To be sure, we still have a great deal to learn about fructose's role in aging, cancer, and the other health issues covered in this chapter. Still, we know plenty about fructose's effect on your weight and risk for heart disease, among several other major threats. Think of the potential benefits described here as added incentives to adopt and stick with a low-fructose lifestyle.

Fructose and Aging

Ad campaigns for soft drinks and other products that are sweetened with large amounts of sugar and high-fructose corn syrup (HFCS) often feature images of youthful, active people. Ironically, consuming too many foods and beverages that contain high concentrations of fructose may actually accelerate aging and overall physical decline.

Although it may taste sweet, fructose is a volatile chemical. When it makes contact with proteins and amino acids in your body, fructose sparks a chemical reaction similar to the one that occurs when you toast bread or roast meat, known as the Maillard reaction. This chemical change produces molecules called advanced glycation end products, or AGEs. As you will see, the abbreviation is disturbingly appropriate.

Normally, your body manufactures AGEs at a slow, steady pace. Certain conditions, however, cause levels of AGEs to increase. Glucose, like fructose, reacts with proteins in the body to produce AGEs. People with poorly controlled diabetes have elevated blood levels of glucose. Not surprisingly, they also tend to have very high concentrations of AGEs, which have been linked to blindness, kidney and nerve damage, and other common diabetes complications.

AGEs damage collagen, the fibrous material that accounts for about 30 percent of the protein in the human body. Collagen is the main component of the connective tissue in tendons, ligaments, organ walls, blood vessels, cartilage, and the inner portion of bones. High activity by AGEs also seems to attract oxidative stress and inflammation.

AGES IN YOUR DIET

Your body produces advanced glycation end products (AGEs), but diet is also a major source of these damaging molecules. As a rule, foods that are high in fat and protein tend to have higher concentrations of AGEs than foods that are primarily carbohydrate. Butter, for example, has 500 times more AGEs by weight than whole wheat bread.

Cooking temperature and duration, among other factors, also influence a food's AGE content. Need another reason to switch from cola to seltzer? The caramel coloring that gives the former its trademark dark hue is a rich source of AGEs.

Many longevity experts believe that AGEs play a critical role in the aging process.

While you have far more glucose circulating in your blood, research suggests that fructose is up to 10 times more efficient at producing AGEs. In one study, Israeli researchers fed water sweetened with fructose, glucose, or sucrose (which is half fructose and half glucose) to different groups of laboratory rats. Over the course of a year, the rats that drank fructose water experienced significantly greater age-related changes in their bones and skin than the rats given glucose or sucrose.

Fructose and Your Brain

Consuming small amounts of fructose may actually sharpen your wits and perk up your brain cells. But some research suggests that a steady diet of high-fructose foods and beverages could have the opposite effect.

As you know, consuming fructose causes the body to produce uric acid. Uric acid can act as an antioxidant, meaning that it protects body tissue from destructive oxidative stress, including your brain. Paradoxically, a 2007 study found that people with elevated uric acid tended to score poorly on tests of cognitive skills.

Researchers at Johns Hopkins University Hospital asked 96 people from the Baltimore area, all between ages 65 and 92, to take a series of tests designed to assess their ability to recall lists of words and names. Next, the Hopkins team measured the volunteers' uric acid levels, revealed by blood tests to be in the range of 1.5 mg/dl to 7.6 mg/dl. The men in this study were deemed to have mildly elevated uric acid if their readings were greater than 5.8 mg/dl; for the women, the benchmark was 4.8 mg/dl. After ruling out the influence of age, education, and other variables, the authors concluded that people with elevated uric acid were up to five times more likely to score below average on memory tests. Using magnetic resonance imaging (MRI), the same group of scientists has also shown that adults 60 and older who have high uric acid are four to five times more likely to have brain changes suggestive of damage to small blood vessels, which may contribute to vascular dementia, the second most common form of dementia after Alzheimer's disease.

Having high uric acid levels in the blood may interfere with mental clarity and processing speed in several ways. A healthy brain requires steady and plentiful blood flow. As I explained in Chapter 5, rising uric acid levels can disrupt circulation by making blood vessels constrict, raising blood pressure. Studies show that people with hypertension are more likely to develop dementia, or the loss of intellectual ability caused by damage to brain cells. What's more, animal studies show that fructose and uric acid injure small blood vessels.

Fructose and Your Joints

Eating a high-fructose diet increases the risk for gout by elevating uric acid levels, as I noted in Chapter 5. Gout affects about 8 of every 1,000 people, according to the National Institute of Arthritis and Musculoskeletal and Skin Diseases. The prime victims are men over age 40; in fact, gout is the most common form of inflammatory arthritis among males. Women under age 50 rarely develop the condition, though their risk rises after menopause; this suggests that hormones provide some protection. In addition to the big toe, gout may produce swelling and inflammation in the elbows, wrists, fingers, knees, and ankles.

For centuries, doctors suspected that consuming certain foods and beverages could trigger this agonizing form of arthritis, but they primarily blamed fatty meats and alcohol. We have known for about 50 years now that fructose raises uric acid, which can form painful crystals in joints. In fact, one study found that a person who eats just one apple or orange per day is 60 percent more likely to develop gout than someone who rarely eats fruit. I'm not suggesting that you should give up fruit for good, but this statistic illustrates the powerful influence of fructose on the risk for gout. Interestingly, according to some estimates, the incidence of gout has doubled in the United States since 1969, a period in which fructose consumption in this country rose by 30 percent.

PAIN AND PRIDE

Gout has been closely associated with men of achievement since early history. In fact, the belief that gout sufferers enjoyed unusual wisdom and leadership qualities was so pervasive that many heroes of Greek mythology were said to have the disease, including King Priam of Troy, Achilles, Odysseus, and Oedipus. The painful condition known to some sufferers as "gouch" was a symbol of status, sometimes referred to as "prosperous gout" or "preeminent gout." In the definitive book on the history of the disease, *Gout: The Patrician Malady,* authors Roy Porter and G. S. Rousseau note that acquiring gout was widely believed to impart wisdom because it "encouraged one to be ruled by one's head not one's feet."

The perception of gout eventually changed, however. By the Colonial era, some viewed the condition as retribution for living a life of luxury and leisure. "Be temperate in wine, in eating, girls, and cloth, or the Gout will seize you and plague you both," wrote Benjamin Franklin, who suffered from the disease and who, according to historical accounts, failed in all respects to heed his own advice.

Fructose and Your Kidneys

Until this point, I haven't spent much time discussing a grave health threat that may arise when you consume too much fructose: kidney disease. We have discovered in recent years that this potentially lethal condition is far more common than we previously realized, affecting over 20 million Americans. Many have only mildly reduced kidney function and will not progress to end-stage renal disease, or kidney failure, which requires dialysis or an organ transplant. However, this is no cause for reassurance; even mild kidney disease can cause high blood pressure and increase the risk for heart disease.

Although we're still studying the issue, it appears likely that the extraordinary amount of fructose in our diets is helping to drive up rates of kidney disease. We know, for instance, that laboratory animals develop kidney disorders if they're fed large amounts of fructose. We also know that existing kidney disease worsens quickly if we feed lab animals diets rich in fructose. (Interestingly, feeding the animals glucose, or starch, has no effect on their kidneys.) We also see a deterioration of kidney disease in lab animals if we raise their uric acid with special enzyme inhibitors. Emerging research involving humans with kidney disease suggests that lowering uric acid with drugs may slow its progression.

Fructose and Your Liver

There is a common perception that liver disease primarily affects people who drink too much alcohol, but this is far from true. In fact, up to 20 percent of Americans have non-alcoholic fatty liver disease (NAFLD), according to the National Institute of Diabetes and Digestive and Kidney Diseases, though rates are much higher among people who

DIET, KIDNEY DISEASE, AND URIC ACID

If you have kidney disease, you may have been instructed to eat a low-protein diet. This recommendation is based on animal studies from the 1980s, which found that reducing dietary protein can slow progression of the disease. Human studies, however, have largely failed to show that low-protein diets prevent worsening of kidney disease.

Recent studies by my group and others may help explain these disappointing results. They suggest that only animal and fish protein—and *not* vegetable protein—damages the kidneys. I suspect one reason could be that animal and fish protein is rich in purines, which raise uric acid. We know from other laboratory-based research that raising uric acid by eating a high-purine diet or by any other means worsens existing kidney disease.

Another reason that low-protein diets may not help kidney disease is that they lead to increased carbohydrate consumption. This could result in eating large amounts of fructose-rich foods, which, of course, will raise uric acid. More research is necessary to determine the ideal diet for people with kidney disease.

are overweight or obese. Though the exact cause of NAFLD is unknown, there is good reason to believe that tossing down too much of another kind of beverage—fructose-sweetened soft drinks—and eating other sugary foods may play a role.

NAFLD is a general term for several conditions caused by the accumulation of fat in liver cells. NAFLD is most common in middle-aged people who are overweight and have other conditions of metabolic syndrome, such as elevated triglycerides and insulin resistance. In fact, developing metabolic syndrome results in a 30-fold increased risk for NAFLD.

Furthermore, though NAFLD was once rare in children, this is no longer true. A 2006 study of people in the San Diego area under age 20 found that about 1 in 10 had NAFLD. Patients with NAFLD can develop scarring of the liver that worsens over time. Eventually, they may develop cirrhosis, which can result in liver failure and death.

Because NAFLD is common in people who have metabolic syndrome, it's reasonable to suspect that a high-fructose diet may contribute to the buildup of fat in the liver—a suspicion supported by science. Feeding fructose to laboratory rats causes their liver cells to fill up with triglycerides. Before long, the rats develop fatty liver.

My colleagues and I have collaborated with Dr. Manal Abdelmalek at Duke University to study the link between fructose and NAFLD. We have found that, compared to people with other forms of liver disease, patients who have NAFLD tend to consume large amounts of fructose, especially from soft drinks. In fact, people with NAFLD consume three times more fructose-rich soft drinks than the average American. We have also discovered that these patients' liver cells have high levels of fructose enzymes—not surprising since a high-fructose diet stimulates these important enzymes. Finally, we

FAST-FOOD INDIGNATION

In the documentary *Super Size Me*, filmmaker Morgan Spurlock eats all of his meals at McDonald's restaurants for 30 days to illustrate the perils of overindulging in fast food. Spurlock gained 25 pounds during his monthlong Big Mac binge, but his physician was most concerned about the damage his patient's experiment was having on one particular body part. Blood tests showed that Spurlock's liver enzymes had soared, a sure sign that the organ was undergoing extreme stress—as if he were drinking excessive amounts of alcohol. "You're pickling your liver!" Spurlock's indignant doctor scolded, imploring him to end his fast-food-only diet or risk long-term harm to his health.

Failing his liver-enzyme test suggests that Spurlock was well on his way to developing full-blown fatty liver (NAFLD), which may progress over time to cirrhosis. Even though he was consuming massive amounts of saturated fat, trans fat, and sodium every day, our studies suggest that it was most likely the extra-large cups of fructose-rich soda that were the cause of his liver problems and posed the swiftest and most serious threat to Spurlock's well-being.

have found that NAFLD patients who take in the most fructose have the worst degree of liver damage.

There is also evidence that raising levels of fructose enzymes by consuming too much sugar and HFCS causes liver damage. One of our collaborators used nuclear magnetic resonance (NMR) spectroscopy to study the livers of patients with NAFLD. NMR can measure the levels of adenosine triphosphate (ATP)—a cell's energy source—in a patient's liver. Using this technique, she was able to show that patients with NAFLD experience a marked drop in liver ATP levels after receiving fructose through an intravenous injection. Even more worrisome, this fall in ATP levels persists for at least 1 hour. By contrast, healthy people experience a drop in liver ATP when infused with fructose, but their levels of stored energy recover quickly.

As you'll recall, cells that become depleted of ATP undergo the phenomenon I call cell shock, meaning they become sickly and weak. These studies suggest that consuming too much fructose is likely the cause of NAFLD.

Fructose and Your Digestive System

Call it the Halloween Hangover: Filling up on sweets often leads to an upset stomach. This is because many people have difficulty digesting the fructose in sugar, HFCS, and other sweeteners. But it's not only candy-munching trick-or-treaters who are affected by this problem, known as fructose malabsorption (or sometimes dietary fructose intolerance). If you have been experiencing unexplained digestive problems, fructose could be the cause.

As fructose travels through the digestive system, it eventually enters the small intestine. From there, it normally is absorbed into the bloodstream. But some people absorb fructose less efficiently than others do. In these cases, fructose enters into the large intestine, where it is broken down by bacteria, producing large amounts of hydrogen gas. Fructose can also suck water into the colon.

Fructose malabsorption causes a variety of gastrointestinal problems, including abdominal pain, bloating, cramps, flatulence, diarrhea, and constipation. Bacteria can convert fructose to compounds called ketoacids; in rare cases, this could cause the blood to become dangerously acidic, a condition that can lead to rapid breathing, confusion, and other symptoms.

In one small 2005 study published in the *Journal of the American Dietetic Association,* researchers asked 15 volunteers to drink water laced with 25 grams of fructose, which is similar to the amount found in a 12-ounce can of nondiet soda. Breath tests that measure hydrogen determined that more than half of the subjects had evidence of fructose malabsorption. Six of the volunteers developed gas or rumbling sounds in their stomachs, and one experienced abdominal pain. When the dose was increased to 50 grams of fructose, breath tests showed that 11 of the 15 volunteers had reached the threshold for fructose malabsorption.

HEREDITARY FRUCTOSE INTOLERANCE

Don't confuse fructose malabsorption or dietary fructose intolerance with a rare condition called hereditary fructose intolerance, or HFI. This genetic disorder occurs in people who are born lacking an enzyme called aldolase B, which helps to convert fructose into energy. Consuming fructose causes people with HFI to experience a severe drop in blood glucose. Over time, they can develop liver damage, too. There is no cure for HFI, so those who have the condition must avoid fruit, sugar, and any other source of fructose. About 1 person in 20,000 is born with HFI.

FRUCTOSE AND STATURE

As I have explained throughout this book, eating too much fructose can make you gain a great deal of weight. Research suggests that children who drink excessive amounts of fructose-rich fruit juice may develop a different sort of problem: They grow too slowly.

A 1997 study by Columbia University researchers found that 2- and 5-year-old children who drink more than 12 ounces of fruit juice per day not only are more likely to be obese, they also are shorter than kids who drink less fruit juice. In fact, the heavy juice drinkers were three times more likely than the other children to be classified as having short stature (defined as being below the 20th percentile in height for sex and age).

One explanation could be that drinking too much fruit juice crowds out another beverage that we know is good for you—milk—as well as other nutritious foods needed for growing bones and muscles. Furthermore, a high-fructose diet interferes with healthy endothelial function, which also is important for growth.

Recent research suggests that fructose may be one cause of irritable bowel syndrome (IBS), a condition that affects up to one in five Americans. Previously, the foods and beverages most commonly linked to IBS were wheat and other grains, chocolate, and dairy products, as well as alcohol. Now studies suggest that many people who complain of IBS symptoms have fructose malabsorption. In a University of Iowa study, for example, more than one-third of people with IBS-like symptoms had dietary fructose intolerance.

If you struggle with gastrointestinal problems, adopting a low-fructose diet may help. A 2006 study published in the *Journal of the American Dietetic Association* found that 74 percent of IBS patients who cut back on their fructose consumption experienced a significant drop in gastrointestinal symptoms.

Fructose and Cancer

Although the evidence is not crystal clear, a number of studies suggest that consuming too much fructose may be a risk factor for certain cancers. For instance, researchers at the Centers for Disease Control and Prevention (CDC) in Atlanta compared the diets of 568 women who had breast cancer with the diets of 1,451 women who were healthy in an attempt to identify foods, ingredients, or eating habits that might increase risk for the disease. The researchers found no connection between breast cancer and the amount of food a woman consumed every day. Red meat did not seem to increase risk, nor did dairy foods or any form of dietary fat.

The CDC team did find that women who consumed sweet foods and beverages roughly 10 times per week were 32 percent more likely to develop early-stage breast cancer than women who avoided high-sugar foods. A similar study of Mexican women correlated an even greater risk for breast cancer with exposure to fructose-rich foods. These and other investigations suggest that reducing fructose intake may complement any steps you are already taking to protect against breast and other common cancers.

For example, a 2005 study by Harvard researchers of more than 130,000 men and women found that males who consumed the most fructose or refined sugar (which is half fructose) had a 37 percent higher risk for colorectal cancer. The Harvard group found no excess risk for colorectal cancer among females, regardless of how much fructose or sugar they consumed. Yet a 2002 Harvard study showed that women tripled their risk for pancreatic cancer if they were overweight, sedentary, and ate a high-fructose diet.

This association was confirmed in a Swedish study of more than 77,000 men and women over age 45. In that study, people who drank two or more sugar-sweetened soft drinks per day had nearly double the risk for pancreatic cancer, which is usually fatal.

Furthermore, we know that a high-fructose diet can cause insulin resistance and elevated insulin, or hyperinsulinemia. In a 2006 study by Mayo Clinic researchers, people with these conditions were at highest risk for developing colon and rectal cancers. Interestingly, the study also showed that elevated blood glucose had only a marginal influence on cancer risk.

As I mentioned, not all studies are correlating high-fructose diets and increased cancer risk. In fact, some research suggests that fructose could have the opposite effect with regard to certain forms of cancer. For example, in a Harvard study of nearly 48,000 male health professionals, the men who consumed the most fructose were half as likely as men who consumed little of the simple sugar to develop advanced prostate cancer. What's most surprising about this finding is that fructose was associated with a lower risk for prostate cancer whether the sugar came from fruit or nonfruit sources. It's not clear why this would be true, and to my knowledge, no one has confirmed the results of this research with a follow-up study.

Clearly, we still have a lot to learn. But if a high-fructose diet *does* cause cancer, then the key question is how. Over the years, science has linked a number of different types of cancer to a natural function of the human body that has run amok: inflammation. Our studies at the University of Florida have revealed that daily dosing with fructose may be stoking low-grade, chronic inflammation, potentially increasing the risk for one of these devastating diseases.

As I explained in Chapter 6, your immune system produces inflammation to help heal wounds and destroy infectious germs. But an overactive and dysfunctional immune system can misfire, attacking healthy tissue and resulting in diseases such as rheumatoid arthritis and lupus erythematosus.

Likewise, persistent inflammation appears to play a role in some cancers. Normally, the body regulates inflammation by turning down the immune system's activity once an injury has healed or an infection is under control. If this regulatory system fails, chronic inflammation may result, causing extensive harm to healthy tissue and organs. In response, the body is forced to continuously repair and rebuild the damaged tissue. With increased cell turnover comes the heightened risk of producing cells with cancer-causing mutations, which could proliferate and form malignant tumors.

We know that certain infections, which cause acute inflammation, can increase the risk for some cancers. For example, human papillomaviruses are a major cause of cervical cancer and have been implicated in other forms of the disease. Moreover, chronic inflammation appears to increase the risk for cancers of the esophagus, lungs, stomach, pancreas, colon, and liver.

The discovery that chronic inflammation may play a part in tumor formation has led us to ask a pertinent question: What's causing this inflammation? We're still studying the question, though our research at the University of Florida clearly showed that exposing human cells to fructose causes them to become highly inflamed. Fructose also

stimulates the production of free radicals, which are responsible for the cellular damage of oxidative stress. And
oxidative stress has itself been implicated as a contributor
to cancer.

Fructose and Your Eyes

Some people with diabetes believe that fructose-sweetened
foods are safe to eat, because they do not raise blood glu-

FRUCTOSE AND PREECLAMPSIA

Eating and drinking too many sugary foods and beverages during pregnancy
may increase the risk for a complication called preeclampsia. Approximately
7 percent of pregnant women develop preeclampsia, which causes high blood
pressure and the loss of large amounts of protein in the urine. Symptoms
include swelling of the face and hands, severe and nonstop headaches, stomach pain, nausea, and disturbed vision. In rare cases, preeclampsia can cause
seizures. Preeclampsia also poses a risk to the fetus, because it often forces
early delivery, which can result in low birth weight. Preeclampsia typically
occurs after the 20th week of a first pregnancy and disappears after delivery.

Ananth Karumanchi, MD, and colleagues at Beth Israel Hospital in Boston have shown that preeclampsia is probably caused by a protein released
from the placenta, which circulates in the blood and injures the endothelial
cells that line blood vessels. Interestingly, elevated uric acid is a characteristic of preeclampsia. As we know, uric acid also causes damage to the endothe-
lium, so it may accelerate and worsen preeclampsia.

Women who develop preeclampsia tend to be overweight and have other
conditions of metabolic syndrome, such as insulin resistance and elevated
blood fats. The combination of overweight, metabolic syndrome, and elevated
uric acid suggests that high-fructose diets may play a role in preeclampsia.

Some evidence supports this theory. In a 2001 study, Norwegian researchers asked 3,133 pregnant women to describe their diets. Women who consumed the most sugar as a percentage of their total calories—especially
sweetened soft drinks—increased their risk for preeclampsia more than
threefold. In particular, women who developed preeclampsia early in their
pregnancies (before the 37th week) drank 22 ounces of soft drinks every day,
on average, compared with about 6 ounces per day for women who did not
develop preeclampsia.

cose levels. This dietary strategy is highly questionable, however, given the many other problems associated with consuming fructose that I have described in these pages. One additional potential threat posed by a high-fructose diet—one of particular concern to people with diabetes—is vision problems, especially cataracts.

Cataracts occur when proteins in the eye undergo changes and form cloudy or opaque areas on the lens. A variety of visual disturbances may result, including "halos," glare, muted colors, loss of night vision, and double vision. Diabetes is a leading cause of cataracts.

Controlling blood glucose levels is the key to preventing common diabetes complications such as vision problems. Some studies suggest that cutting back on fructose may be critical, too. In one study, Canadian researchers fed diabetic rats one of two dietary regimens—glucose and cornstarch or fructose and cornstarch. Using laser scanners, the researchers examined the rats' eyes after several months. They found that the rats given fructose were more likely to develop cataracts.

Fructose and Your Teeth

In the United States, children today have more cavities than children of the late 1980s and early 1990s, according to a 2007 report by the CDC. In fact, tooth decay had been declining for decades, thanks to public education and the introduction of dental products containing fluoride. But the CDC determined that 28 percent of preschoolers have at least one cavity in their baby teeth, up from 24 percent during the period from 1988 to 1994.

The CDC study did not set out to identify the reasons for this unwelcome trend in children's oral health. Most dentists say that the rising consumption of soda and fruit juice is at least partly to blame.

Fructose is a carbohydrate, and the bacteria in your mouth thrive on all carbs, both sugars and starches. As bacteria feed on carbohydrates, they produce acids that eat away at your teeth's protective enamel. If you consume lots of carbohydrates but don't brush and floss regularly, you end up spending a lot of time in the dentist's chair. Studies have shown that people (especially children) who drink the most soda, fruit juice, and other fructose-sweetened beverages are at significantly higher risk for developing cavities.

You have probably been hearing some version of what you just read from your dentist since you were a child. But soda is even worse for your teeth than you may have realized, whether or not it contains fructose. Most carbonated soft drinks, both diet and nondiet, contain phosphoric acid and/or citric acid, which can erode dental enamel, too.

A 2007 study in *General Dentistry* measured the pH of a number of different soft drinks and found that almost all of them were highly acidic. In fact, some colas approached the acidity of battery acid. Other studies have shown that orange juice and sports drinks, which also tend to be acidic, can reduce the surface hardness of teeth.

If you want to protect your teeth *and* limit your fructose—but you simply must drink something sweet tasting and carbonated—the best choice may be diet root beer. The reason: It doesn't contain large amounts of the acids found in colas and other types of sodas.

Some dentists advise patients to gulp down sweetened soft drinks quickly instead of drinking them in a leisurely way to ensure that their teeth are not bathed in sugary liquid for a prolonged period. As I explained in an earlier chapter, rapidly consuming beverages that contain a large amount of sugar or HFCS can cause your blood fructose levels to soar, which results in worse metabolic damage. Instead of chugging a soft drink, spare your teeth some damage by slowly sipping with a straw.

PART III

SWEET SALVATION: THE LOW-FRUCTOSE SOLUTION

CHAPTER 8

STEAK AND POTATOES

Why We Need a New Approach to Weight Loss

Which one of these foods is worse for your waistline and heart: a juicy slab of prime rib or a plain baked potato served on the side?

A generation ago, that question would have seemed absurd. Research had linked diets high in fat and cholesterol to an increased risk for heart attack and stroke. Doctors issued strict mandates to their patients: Cut back on steaks, eggs, and butter; eat more carbohydrates.

Many people took this dietary directive as an invitation to fill up on starchy foods such as potatoes, bread, pasta, and rice. But in recent years, the authors of many weight-loss plans have demonized carbohydrates as the true cause of obesity, type 2 diabetes, and heart disease. They point out that the percentage of Americans who are overweight has soared since the dawn of the low-fat era. If you dine out with a friend who orders a hamburger—hold the bun—you can be sure that he or she is on a low-carb diet.

So who is right? What's the best dietary approach to weight loss and optimal health—low carb or low fat? The steak or the potato?

Scientists are still trying to sort out the relative benefits of low-fat and low-carb diets. In my view, there are flaws in both approaches.

Although fructose is a carbohydrate, the Low-Fructose Diet is *not* another low-carb eating plan. As I will explain in the pages to come, there is no reason to dramatically restrict all carbohydrates in your diet, because they are not created equal. Some carbs are good for you, while others are not. Fructose is probably the worst of all.

People who try low-carb diets often complain that they miss certain foods, such as baked potatoes, as well as bread, rice, and other starches. Low-carb diets banish or severely limit starches because they are formed by long chains of glucose. This simple sugar, according to low-carb proponents, is a major menace. Eating starchy foods, they point out, causes a rapid rise in blood sugar, which they blame for all sorts of metabolic problems.

If you have tried a low-carb diet and found yourself craving potatoes, rice, and bread, then you will be pleasantly surprised to learn that the Low-Fructose Diet does not prohibit these or other starches. There is simply no reason to. Glucose is not the problem. Fructose is.

The scientific literature is quite clear on this point. As I have explained in the preceding chapters, fructose is unique in its ability to trigger the following metabolic changes that cause weight gain, damage the cardiovascular system, and set the stage for diabetes.

- Metabolizing fructose forces cells to burn up adenosine triphosphate, their energy "currency," too quickly.

- Fructose causes uric acid to rise.

- Fructose contributes to insulin resistance and leptin resistance.

- Fructose causes inflammation and oxidative stress.

By contrast, glucose is capable of triggering these harmful metabolic changes only under certain circumstances—namely, if a person has full-blown diabetes. For everyone else, dietary glucose does not present any serious problems. I believe that the various creators of today's most widely used weight-loss plans made important strides in our understanding of the best way to eat for optimal health. I also believe that by focusing on glucose, they target some foods inappropriately while failing to adequately address the real problem: fructose.

If you have another diet book on your bookshelf, chances are that it may include only a brief reference to fructose, if any at all. In the following pages, I will discuss the benefits and shortcomings of the major diet strategies of the past generation, with an emphasis on how they fail to account for the fructose factor.

A caveat: As anyone who has ever browsed the "diet and nutrition" shelf of a bookstore or library knows, diet books offer a stunning assortment of slimming strategies and theories. For example, one popular diet recommends choosing foods according to your blood type. Another suggests limiting the variety of flavors in individual meals to prevent "appetite meters" in the brain from becoming overstimulated, causing you to eat too much. If you are old enough, you may recall the infamous "martinis and whipped cream" diet that was briefly popular in the 1960s.

I have made no attempt to include an exhaustive analysis of every diet developed in recent memory. Instead, this chapter focuses on the three major nutritional approaches of the past generation or so: the low-fat diet, the low-carb diet, and the low-glycemic diet.

The Low-Fat Diet

People of a certain age may recall a time when no one worried about fat in the diet. A pork chop or a thick slice of meat loaf was considered a wholesome dinner. Everybody drank whole milk and slathered butter on their toast without giving it a second thought. Low-fat cookies, cakes, and potato chips were unheard of.

That all changed, thanks largely to the work of a University of Minnesota physiologist and nutritionist named Ancel Keys, PhD (1904–2004). A half-century ago, Dr. Keys was one of the first scientists to suggest that eating too much fat was unhealthy. Today, the USDA, the American Heart Association, the American Diabetes Association, and virtually all major public health organizations that offer advice about what to eat recommend some version of a low-fat diet.

To be sure, no nutrition scientist has had a greater influence on the American diet than Dr. Keys. After World War II, he became interested in the link between heart disease and diet when he noticed a pair of surprising trends. American business executives, who could afford to eat whatever they liked, were having an alarming number of heart attacks. Meanwhile, rates of cardiovascular disease were plummeting in parts of Europe that were experiencing severe postwar food shortages.

Puzzled by this apparent contradiction, Dr. Keys and several colleagues decided to track the diets and death rates from cardiovascular disease among people in various countries around the world. The study found a clear link: People who ate a lot of fatty foods were at high risk for fatal heart attacks and strokes. The link between animal fat, in particular, and cardiovascular disease appeared to be linear; that is, the more you eat, the higher your risk is.

It's impossible to overstate the impact of Dr. Keys's work. Still, he had critics practically from the start. For instance, Dr. Keys's initial study included six countries. Yet several skeptics pointed out that at the time, data on fat consumption and heart disease were available from more than 20 countries. Including all of the data, critics charged, would make the link between dietary fat and heart disease look less convincing.

What's more, Dr. Keys's antifat message was translated to the public in a way that made *all* forms of fat seem unhealthy, which we now know is not true. A few small trials have shown some benefit to dramatically limiting overall fat intake. For example, Dean Ornish, MD, the author of several popular diet books, published a paper in a 1990 issue of the British medical journal *Lancet* in which he reported that patients with cardiovascular disease who adopted an extremely low-fat diet were able to reduce the amount of plaque in their arteries.

More recent studies comparing different types of diets have produced striking evidence that cutting back on all fat

A RATION-AL WAY TO EAT

Ancel Keys, PhD, is known as the father of the low-fat diet, but his first major achievement as a nutritionist came during World War II. The US Department of Defense asked Dr. Keys to come up with a way to provide combat soldiers with nonperishable, balanced meals they could carry on the battlefield. His solution: ready-to-eat provisions called Field Rations, Type K, which eventually came to be known as K rations or K rats. A typical supper unit included a tin of canned meat, biscuits, candy, chewing gum, and cigarettes.

does not prevent heart attacks, nor is it necessarily the best way to lose weight. One noteworthy example is the large, federally funded study called the Women's Health Initiative (WHI), which divided more than 48,000 female participants into two groups. About 40 percent of the women were asked to reduce their overall fat intake, while the remainder ate their normal diets.

Researchers tracked both groups for 8 years before publishing their startling findings in a 2006 issue of the *Journal of the American Medical Association*. Among the results? Women who had adopted the low-fat diet suffered just as many heart attacks and strokes as women who had maintained their normal diets. One explanation for the lack of protection from heart disease may be that women in the low-fat group reduced their intake of all fats, including sources of heart-healthy omega-3 fatty acids (such as fatty fish) and monounsaturated fats (such as olive oil and nuts).

A month earlier, *JAMA* had published another paper based on the WHI study showing that women who ate a low-fat diet lost more weight over a 7-year period than their nondieting counterparts—though not much more. After 1 year, women in the low-fat group had lost about

4 pounds extra, on average, compared with women in the control group. After 7 years, the difference in average weight loss between women in the two groups was less than 1 pound. In other words, the low-fat diet prevented weight gain, but it failed to help the women lose weight for an extended period.

Bottom line: While some people who adopt a low-fat eating plan shed pounds, many struggle with maintaining weight loss. The problem may be that low-fat diets have a built-in flaw: Cutting fat from the menu often leads to eating more carbohydrates, which may increase exposure to fructose.

The Low-Carb Diet

Low-carbohydrate diets have been popular for much of the past generation, but they are hardly a new idea. The strategy of eliminating carbohydrate-rich foods to lose weight has gone in and out of fashion since at least the mid-19th century. Low-carb regimens often call for extreme measures. A typical plan might require dieters to drastically reduce their carb intakes for the first 2 weeks by avoiding all fruit, bread and other grains, and starchy vegetables and tubers (such as potatoes). The goal of this strategy is simple: Deprive your body of its preferred fuel source—carbohydrates—and force your cells to produce energy by burning stored fat instead. As your carb-starved body burns fat, byproducts called ketones spill into your blood. Over time, ketones accumulate in your body, creating a condition called ketosis. Proponents of low-carb diets believe that ketosis is good news, a sign that the diet is working. As a physician, I can't say there's much to celebrate about ketosis. At a minimum, ketosis can be an embarrassing nuisance, because ketones may leave your breath smelling strange and fruity. Worse, ketones make the blood acidic, which in extreme cases could result in a condition called ketoacidosis. This unpleasant state causes extreme thirst, nausea, and vomiting.

Ketosis can also interfere with healthy heart function and respiration and lead to the breakdown of muscle tissue. It typically strikes people with undiagnosed diabetes, whose bodies are unable to burn glucose, so they revert to burning fat for energy. There have been reports in the medical literature of ketoacidosis occurring in people who have adopted low-carb diets.

I'm also concerned about the emphasis on fat and protein in many of these diets. Some urge dieters to eat eggs and red meat until they feel satisfied, with no limits on portion size. Yet it's well-known that eating large amounts of animal fat raises blood cholesterol levels. In fact, a 2007 study published in the *Journal of the Medical Association* (*JAMA*) found that people who went on the Atkins diet, perhaps the best known of the low-carb eating plans, experienced a slight rise in LDL ("bad") cholesterol. This increase was all the more worrisome because the dieters had lost a significant amount of weight—which should have *lowered* their cholesterol levels.

Furthermore, as a physician and scientist who specializes in the study and treatment of kidney disease, I am worried about the amount of protein that people may consume on a low-carb diet. Over time, eating too much protein could damage these filtering organs, especially if you already have kidney disease. Unfortunately, mild kidney disease is very common among people who are overweight and have other conditions of metabolic syndrome. It can be present for years before it is diagnosed.

Apart from the medical concerns, the most obvious problem you may face with a low-carb diet is staying on it. This might seem crazy; after all, how could anyone have trouble sticking with a diet that allows for steak, butter, and cheese? But the diet's emphasis on fat and protein, and its near-elimination of carbohydrates, will seem foreign and unusual to many palates, with good reason.

For the past 10,000 years, humans have eaten diets that consist primarily of carbohydrates—typically, anywhere from 40 to 60 percent of calories—with lesser amounts of fat and protein. Major scientific bodies, such as the National Academy of Sciences, recommend choosing diets that derive 45 to 65 percent of calories from carbohydrates. The human body simply seems to run better when carbohydrates are the primary fuel source. Diets that radically reduce carbohydrates are difficult to maintain, so many people who adopt them ultimately relapse, and their weight returns.

Despite my reservations about low-carb diets, I nonetheless believe that they represent a major breakthrough in our approach to treating obesity and metabolic syndrome. Indeed, in head-to-head comparisons with other weight-loss plans, low-carb diets have proven superior. Now research suggests that these diets work because they reduce your intake of one carbohydrate in particular: fructose.

Consider the findings of the 2007 *JAMA* study I mentioned earlier. Stanford researchers placed more than 300 overweight volunteer subjects on one of four different weight-loss plans: the Atkins diet, the Zone diet (a low-carb, high-protein plan), the LEARN diet (a low-fat plan), or the Ornish diet (a very low-fat plan). After 1 year, the volunteers on the Atkins diet maintained a weight loss of about 10 pounds, on average. That's roughly twice as much weight loss as the other volunteers achieved in the same time frame. Interestingly, members of the Atkins group also showed marked improvements in their blood pressure, triglycerides, and HDL cholesterol (the "good" kind). All these benefits accrue when you reduce the amount of fructose in your diet.

Proponents of low-carb diets seem to recognize the value of cutting back on sugar, fruit, and other sources of fructose. Unfortunately, they punish dieters by forbidding other important carbohydrates—in the form of bread, potatoes, and other starchy foods—and encouraging them to eat dangerously large amounts of fat and protein.

Many low-carb diets offer another important, if unintentional, benefit. Let me explain what I mean. The initial 2-week "induction" phase common among these diets dramatically limits your intake of carbohydrates to less than 20 grams per day. As I explained earlier, the goal of removing carbs from the diet is to induce a state of ketosis, during which the body burns fat for energy.

The true benefit of this 2-week ultra-low-carb phase lies elsewhere. Specifically, it gives your body a vacation from the worst carbohydrate of all: fructose. As a result, your fructose enzymes plunge. These enzymes are responsible for processing fructose, which generates uric acid, drains energy from cells, and produces other unhealthy metabolic changes that result in weight gain and other problems.

When you eat fructose, levels of fructose enzymes rise. If you eat a lot of fructose, you may have very high levels of

STEAK AND POTATOES   157

THE ORIGINAL LOW-CARB MAN

Robert Atkins, MD, was a polarizing figure in the weight-loss world. But he did not create the first low-carb diet. This distinction probably belongs to a London undertaker named William Banting, whose best-selling 1864 book *Letter on Corpulence* described how he lost 50 pounds "and nearly 13 inches in bulk" by eating mutton, fish, and other high-protein foods while avoiding most carbohydrates. Thanks to the popularity of *Letter on Corpulence,* the high-protein, low-carb approach to weight loss came to be known as bantingism.

these enzymes, which can rise two- to threefold higher than normal in some people, according to our research. As your fructose enzymes climb, each serving of fructose becomes more toxic.

Elevated fructose enzymes make weight loss more difficult. On the other hand, studies have shown that a 2-week fructose-free diet can reverse this problem and restore fructose enzymes to normal levels. Once these enzymes are under control, eating modest servings of fruit and other fructose-rich foods will help you stay healthy.

Through a bit of serendipity, the 2-week carb-free phase that kicks off most low-carb diets turns out to be just what many people need to bring their fructose enzymes back in line. As I will explain in Chapter 11, my diet allows you to enjoy the benefits of lower fructose enzymes without forcing your body into an unhealthy state of ketosis. Eating reasonable servings of the very foods that are commonly forbidden for the first 2 weeks of most low-carb diets—bread and other starchy glucose-rich foods—will keep you from getting sick.

The Low-Glycemic Diet

In a sense, the low-glycemic diet represents a compromise between low-fat and low-carb diets. These plans tend to discourage eating large amounts of red meat, whole-fat dairy foods, and other sources of saturated fat. Instead, they typically encourage dieters to consume plenty of "good" fats—such as olive oil and fatty fish—which help satisfy appetite and appear to lower the risk for heart disease. More important, low-glycemic diets do not drastically limit all carbohydrates. Instead, they encourage dieters to choose "good" carbs and avoid "bad" ones by using a rating scale called the glycemic index.

The word *glycemia* refers to the presence of glucose in the blood. In the late 1970s, researchers at the University of Toronto developed the glycemic index as a method for predicting how much a food containing carbohydrates raises blood glucose, also called blood sugar. During digestion, carbohydrates break down to glucose and enter the bloodstream. Some carbs produce a steep and rapid rise in blood glucose levels, while others have a more gradual effect.

David Jenkins, MD, and his team created the glycemic index as a tool to help diabetes patients. Normally, when a person consumes carbohydrates, the pancreas responds by producing insulin. This hormone acts as a gatekeeper, allowing glucose to enter cells in organs throughout the body, where it is stored or burned as energy. In people with diabetes, either the pancreas isn't able to produce insulin or the insulin doesn't work as it should. Many rely on medication and careful meal planning to help their bodies use glucose as energy and prevent blood sugar from rising too high and damaging organs.

The glycemic index, or GI, allows people with diabetes to limit or avoid carbohydrates that will strain their capacity to control their blood sugar levels (high-GI foods) while favoring others that will be less taxing (low-GI foods). Using this strategy makes sense for people who have diabetes, for whom large swings in blood sugar are unhealthy and may cause a variety of both short- and long-term complications.

In general, sweet and starchy foods have moderate to high GI rankings. According to proponents of low-glycemic diets, avoiding these foods will speed up weight loss and prevent metabolic syndrome. They portray insulin as a key player in weight gain. High-GI foods overstimulate the pancreas, causing it to produce large amounts of the hormone. As a result, insulin overwhelms glucose and ends up removing too much of it from the blood. So eating high-GI foods causes blood sugar to soar, only to come crashing down. Soon after eating a large serving of high-GI foods,

---

THE GLYCEMIC INDEX: A SNAPSHOT

The glycemic index (GI) ranks foods according to how rapidly they cause blood glucose levels to rise on a scale of 0 to 100 or higher. Proponents say that eating low-GI foods promotes weight loss and prevents diabetes, heart disease, and other conditions. Here are the rankings of some common foods.

	TYPICAL FOODS
Low-GI foods (below 55)	Apples, beans, corn, oranges, milk, chocolate bars
Moderate-GI foods (55 to 70)	Pancakes, macaroni and cheese, table sugar, honey, beer
High-GI foods (above 70)	Baked potatoes, rice, cornflakes, white bread, jelly beans

Source: The New Glucose Revolution (Marlowe & Company, 2007)

As you can see, the glycemic index favorably ranks some foods that are very high in sugar, such as fruit and candy. This can occur because other elements in a food, such as fat or fiber, can slow down digestion, which blunts the rise in blood glucose after you consume carbohydrates such as sugar. But fat and fiber do not prevent the fructose in sugary foods from "shocking" cells, causing a rise in uric acid and other metabolic problems.

you become hungry and want to eat again—especially craving carbohydrates.

And so begins a vicious cycle caused by eating high-GI foods, which overstimulate the pancreas. It's an interesting theory, but it is not well supported by the metabolic facts. Stimulating the pancreas to produce insulin is not the problem. Your body is *supposed* to produce insulin when blood glucose levels rise, so that's normal and healthy. It is insulin resistance that is closely linked to metabolic syndrome and weight gain. Glucose does not cause insulin resistance. Fructose does. Glucose does not trick your body into persistent hunger. Fructose does.

Because it is half glucose, sugar has a moderately high GI ranking. Accordingly, the low-glycemic diets restrict sugary foods, including fruit, which has the benefit of also restricting the amount of fructose you consume. In my opinion, it is for this reason that low-glycemic diets can help you lose weight and control conditions of metabolic syndrome. What's more, some popular versions of this diet recommend a 2-week induction phase, during which only small servings of carbohydrates are allowed. During that time, a dieter will consume little or no fructose, which restores fructose enzymes to healthy levels.

MY PROBLEM WITH THE GLYCEMIC INDEX

Unless you have diabetes, I don't believe that the glycemic index (GI) has a useful role in choosing foods that will help you lose weight and control conditions such as metabolic syndrome. The GI ranks carbohydrates on a scale of 0 to 100 (or higher, in some cases) according to their effect on blood glucose. High-GI foods, such as potatoes and white bread, cause a steep and rapid rise in blood glucose; low-GI foods, such as beans and oat bread, produce a more modest increase.

The pancreas produces insulin to lower rising blood glucose levels. But eating foods that stimulate insulin production isn't a problem unless you have diabetes. Limiting consumption of foods that induce insulin resistance is of far greater concern. After all, it is insulin resistance—and not the release of insulin by the pancreas—that is linked to obesity, elevated blood fats, and hypertension, as well as the increased risk for diabetes, cardiovascular complications, and kidney disease that accompanies these conditions.

Fructose has a low GI ranking (20), because it does not stimulate the pancreas to release large amounts of insulin. This may give the false impression that choosing foods that are high in fructose can help to prevent diabetes. In fact, we know from laboratory studies that fructose induces insulin resistance and other conditions of metabolic syndrome. Meanwhile, feeding pure glucose to laboratory animals causes a rise in blood glucose levels, but it does not produce insulin resistance.

I believe the glycemic index may be a useful tool for people who have diabetes, which is the population for whom it was initially developed. All patients with type 1 diabetes, and a large number with type 2 diabetes, must take medications (such as injected insulin) in order to maintain safe and healthy blood glucose levels. Most doctors instruct people who are diabetic to limit the total grams of carbohydrate in a meal in order to keep blood glucose from rising too high. High-GI foods raise blood glucose more than equal-size portions of low-GI foods, so using the glycemic index may help people with diabetes fine-tune their meal planning. Nonetheless, the American Diabetes Association recommends using carbohydrate counting as the primary means for controlling blood glucose levels.

CHAPTER 9

GROUP THERAPY

The Major Food Groups
and the Low-Fructose Diet

By now you're probably wondering: What should I eat? We're almost there! Chapter 11 describes the Low-Fructose Diet in detail.

I believe you will find the basic rules of my eating plan to be simple and easy to follow. That said, you may find certain elements puzzling at first. After all, some things I recommend defy conventional wisdom about weight loss. Others may seem like sacrilege, at odds with the tenets of nutrition you have known since you were a child. For instance, if you adhere to the old "apple a day" advice, you will need to set it aside.

To be sure, certain of my diet's principles will sound familiar. But as new research reveals, they may help you lose weight and protect your health for reasons that surprise you.

In short, this chapter anticipates the questions you may

have about the Low-Fructose Diet. Among other things, I'll explain:

- Why fruit is off limits, at least temporarily

- Why you need to limit certain types of vegetables for a short time, too

- Why you can eat many of the starches that low-carb diets condemn, though you'll need to put some thought into which daily bread (and other grains) you choose

- Why something as trivial-seeming as using the wrong sandwich condiment could throw off your diet

This chapter will address these and other issues by offering an overview of the major food groups and how they fit into the Low-Fructose Diet.

Fruit

Fruit poses a dilemma. On the one hand, biting into a crisp apple or a juicy orange slice makes us feel virtuous for a reason. Fruit is full of vitamins and minerals, as well as micronutrients called phytochemicals, which growing scientific evidence suggests can fight disease and aging. Fruit is also an excellent source of fiber. Yet the sweetness that makes apples and oranges so delicious has a bitter edge, because every bite of fruit provides a potent dose of fructose—between 5 and 10 grams per serving, in most cases.

This makes fruit a good news/bad news food group. The large amounts of fructose in fruit activate the unhealthy metabolic pathways I've described in preceding chapters, ultimately causing cells to absorb too much fat and become insulin resistant. On the other hand, the nutrients in fruit—especially vitamin C and potassium—block many of these same pathways.

Because of these opposing influences, a slender, active person may be able to eat fruit without worry. But if you are currently overweight and sedentary, your fructose enzymes—which produce this simple sugar's dangerous effects—are probably raging out of control. If that's the case, any benefits from vitamin C and other nutrients will be trumped by the overwhelming damage that fructose will cause.

You probably never dreamed that a physician would tell you to stop eating fruit, but that's exactly what I'm advising—but only for 2 weeks. During the initial 14-day phase of the Low-Fructose Diet, you will dramatically reduce your fructose intake in order to rein in your fructose enzymes. Abstaining from fruit and other sources of fructose for a brief period will help bring your levels of these enzymes back down to normal and turn off the mechanisms that inflict so much harm. (By the way, this directive also applies to fruit juice, which contains even higher concentrations of fructose than the fruit itself.)

Don't worry—going a couple of weeks without eating fruit is not a threat to your long-term health. To the contrary, this short break from consuming fructose will help to correct metabolic problems that may build up flab, raise your blood pressure, and create other unhealthy symptoms. Besides, unlike low-carbohydrate diets, my plan allows you to eat a variety of vegetables, even during the 2-week introduction, so you will still be consuming natural sources of vitamins, minerals, and phytochemicals.

A REASON TO CHERISH THE CHERRY

To help keep uric acid levels under control, consider taking a cue from gout sufferers, many of whom rely on a secret weapon in the battle against this unusually painful form of arthritis: cherries and cherry juice.

Gout occurs when uric acid forms crystals in the joints. Many drugs for gout focus on lowering uric acid levels. Because fructose raises uric acid, eating any kind of fruit might seem like a good way to trigger an attack of gout, not prevent the problem. Yet cherries may help to do just that.

Researchers at the University of California, Davis, asked 10 healthy women to eat a large serving of pitted Bing cherries—280 grams, or about 45 cherries each. Blood tests conducted 5 hours later showed that the women's uric acid levels had dropped 14.5 percent, on average. When researchers repeated the test with other fruits, none lowered uric acid levels.

Interestingly, uric acid wasn't the only blood element that fell among the women asked to eat cherries. A test for the marker known as C-reactive protein (CRP) showed that the women had slightly less inflammation in their arteries, too. This benefit may be directly linked to cherries' effect on uric acid. Our research shows that rising uric acid stimulates production of CRP in vascular cells. What's more, cherries contain antioxidants, particularly compounds known as anthocyanins, which may reduce inflammation.

We aren't sure how cherries lower uric acid, but it may be that they increase the amount that's excreted by the kidneys. Because a serving of cherries (roughly 10 cherries) contains a modest 4 grams of fructose, snacking on the ruby red fruit is a good way to spend your fructose allowance.

Once you have completed the first phase of the diet, you are free to enjoy fruit and its considerable health benefits once again, but only in moderation and always ensuring that your total fructose intake does not exceed the generous range of 25 to 35 grams per day. Bear in mind that fruit varies greatly in its fructose content. A single plum has just 2 grams of fructose, for example, while a cup of watermelon contains 24 grams, or nearly 1 day's worth.

Eating a variety of fruits is a great idea, as long as they fit into your daily fructose budget. Those with high concentrations of vitamin C may be the best choices, given how effectively this antioxidant nutrient helps to control certain conditions of metabolic syndrome. For instance, we know that people with high blood pressure tend to have low vitamin C levels. Some studies have shown that vitamin C supplements lower blood pressure in certain circumstances. One reason may be that vitamin C promotes healthy endothelial function—that is, it encourages blood vessels to dilate, which in turn promotes good circulation.

Recent studies also have shown that vitamin C may lower blood levels of uric acid by increasing the amount of this troublesome compound that gets excreted in the urine.

Vegetables and Legumes

Diet plans often lump fruits and vegetables into one group, with the usual advice to eat at least five servings per day. But fruits and vegetables are two very different foods. Among their many differences, of course, is the fact that vegetables contain far less fructose than fruits do. Think of vegetables as fruit with all the benefits, but little of the risk.

The benefits of eating vegetables are beyond dispute. Consider what we have known for many years about vegetarians, who—although they are free to eat fruit—usually replace animal protein in their diets with larger servings of vegetables and legumes (which include peas, beans, and lentils). A study of German monks in the 1930s, for example, found that the vegetarians among the men had lower blood pressure and fewer heart attacks than those who ate meat. Many studies have since confirmed the benefits of a vegetarian diet.

The Low-Fructose Diet is by no means vegetarian, but vegetables do play an important role. Eating plenty of produce will promote weight loss and heart health by crowding out foods that are high in fructose, as well as saturated fat and cholesterol. There are some important considerations when selecting vegetables, however. For starters, while few vegetables are overtly sweet, a handful have modestly high levels of fructose. For instance, peas contain more fructose by weight than raspberries. To keep your overall sugar intake as low as possible during the diet's 2-week introduction phase, I primarily recommend vegetables with low fructose concentrations.

Surprisingly, some vegetables, including asparagus, mushrooms, and cauliflower, contain moderately high levels of purines. The same is true of peas, beans, and other legumes. Many gout sufferers avoid these vegetables and

---

A FEW WORDS ABOUT POTATOES

Former low-carb dieters who miss potatoes can rejoice: The Low-Fructose Diet does not forbid the popular spud, or any other tuber. Still, it's important to keep a couple of things in mind.

- Though most varieties of potato contain relatively modest amounts of fructose, the typical 5-inch sweet potato has about 2.6 grams. That's much less than most types of fruit, but it still represents a small portion of your daily fructose budget, so it's worth bearing that in mind in order to keep your overall intake under control. Sweet potatoes are an excellent source of vitamin A, as well as vitamin C, so they may offer some nutritional advantages over plain baked potatoes. But these benefits will be offset if you top a sweet potato with fructose-rich brown sugar, as some recipes recommend.

- Speaking of baked potatoes, smothering one with butter and sour cream adds calories and saturated fat. Likewise, french fries—America's favorite way to eat potatoes—are full of fat and do not qualify as health food simply because they lack fructose and purines. Eat them rarely, if at all, in small servings.

legumes, assuming that their relatively elevated purine content will cause a rise in blood levels of uric acid, leading to a painful arthritic flare-up.

I don't think it's necessary to skip these otherwise healthy foods. A large study of gout patients found no evidence that eating high-purine vegetables increased the risk for a flare-up, probably because people tend to eat these particular vegetables in modest portions. This suggests that they don't cause a steep rise in uric acid, so there's no reason you should avoid them. On the other hand, if you are in the habit of eating asparagus or any other type of high-purine produce every night with dinner, then it's probably a good idea to limit yourself to no more than one or two servings of that vegetable per week.

Bread, Pasta, Rice, and Other Grains

It's true: The Low-Fructose Diet allows you to eat bread, potatoes, rice, and other starchy foods made from grains. This may come as a shock to anyone who has ever been on a low-carb diet, which is based on the principle that eating even modest amounts of starch makes you fat. But this is simply not the case for most people. If you lost weight by following one of these plans, it was probably because you cut back on a different carbohydrate—fructose—which tricks you into being hungry all the time and causes other metabolic problems by raising uric acid.

Grains do not contain fructose, so they do not raise uric acid. But food manufacturers often add sugar, high-fructose corn syrup (HFCS), honey, and other fructose-rich sweeteners to grain products—bread, in particular—to enhance their flavor and appearance. In order to avoid hidden sources of fructose in your diet, read product labels before you buy.

I am going to recommend specific types of bread you can eat during the introductory phase of my diet. As a general rule, keep your fructose intake from bread and related products (such as bagels and English muffins) to a minimum by purchasing varieties that contain no more than 2 or 3 grams of sugar per serving. Some, such as raisin bread, can have up to 6 grams per slice. (The number of grams of sugar per serving is listed on the Nutrition Facts panel, which accompanies the ingredients list.)

There are many different types of bread, of course—enough to fill an entire aisle at most supermarkets. As a rule, the dark, chewy loaves made from whole wheat, oats, and other whole grains contain more healthful fiber than white bread. Studies show that people who consume plenty of whole grains—not just breads but other foods, such as whole wheat pasta and brown rice—tend to have low rates of heart disease and diabetes. That said, during the first phase of my diet, I am going to recommend avoiding certain types of whole grain bread, because many brands contain relatively large amounts of sugar or HFCS. (Rye bread, which rarely contains added fructose, is an excellent choice.)

Pasta does not contain fructose, but tomato-based sauces often do, usually in the form of HFCS. Likewise, the wheat, oats, and other grains used to make breakfast cereal are free of fructose, but these popular products are often coated with sugar. Don't be tricked into thinking that "natural"-sounding breakfast foods are necessarily fructose free; a bowl of granola can contain more sugar than a bowl of Lucky Charms.

Of course, you can turn a simple slice of bread into little more than a vehicle for fructose by slathering it with sugary jelly. Many popular brands of peanut butter are sweetened with sugar, too. Avoid them, but don't despair. Most supermarkets today carry several brands that contain nothing but delicious ground peanuts and a little salt (though unsalted varieties are available, too).

I do not recommend low-carb breads. Taste a slice, and you will see why. These products hit the market in response to the low-carb diet craze. But they offer little advantage if you're on the Low-Fructose Diet, and even less flavor.

Meat and Poultry

Foods that cause gout should be on your diet radar, because they raise uric acid. As this goes, there is strong scientific evidence to suggest that eating too much meat causes gout. Doctors have known this anecdotally for many years. An early 19th-century medical text identified one cause of gout as a "full diet, especially of animal food. . . ."

This long-held suspicion was validated when rheumatologist Hyon K. Choi, MD, of Massachusetts General Hospital and his colleagues analyzed the medical and dietary histories of more than 47,000 men. Over a 12-year period, 730 of the men developed gout, suggesting that they had high uric acid levels. Dr. Choi and his team found that heavy meat eaters had a 41 percent increase in gout risk.

In another study, Dr. Choi and his colleagues showed that the uric acid levels of people who eat the most meat are nearly 0.5 mg/dl higher, on average, than those of people who eat little or no meat. (One study found that every 1 mg/dl rise in uric acid correlates to a 32 percent increase in heart disease risk.)

Meat raises uric acid because it contains purines. Organ meats, such as liver and kidneys, have the highest purine levels. If you enjoy organ meats, eat them no more than once a month (and consider cutting them out altogether). The most popular and widely consumed cuts of beef, pork, and lamb have moderate purine levels. I recommend limiting your consumption of red meat to two or three servings per week. On the other hand, chicken and turkey have lower purine levels, so you can eat poultry more often.

Fish and Seafood

Some fish and shellfish contain large amounts of purines as well, which means that eating them can raise uric acid. But seafood offers tremendous health benefits, too, so it should be a regular feature of your weekly menus.

We have known for decades that fish protects the heart, ever since Danish researchers discovered that a group of Eskimos in Greenland—who ate diets consisting largely of marine foods—rarely suffered heart attacks. Fish oil is one of nature's richest sources of omega-3 fatty acids, which help to regulate heart rhythm. One large study, involving more than 20,000 men, determined that eating just one serving of fish per week reduces the risk of sudden cardiac death— which kills a quarter of a million Americans each year—by about 50 percent. Omega-3 fatty acids appear to confer other benefits, too, such as reducing inflammation.

If you eat a lot of seafood, you may raise your uric acid level. But the effect is not nearly as powerful as the rise in uric acid caused by eating too much meat. A national survey found that the difference in uric acid between the most devoted seafood lovers and those who avoid fish is modest—0.16 mg/dl, on average.

You can further minimize the effect of eating seafood by limiting varieties that are relatively high in purines, according to the guidelines I will present in Chapter 11. This should not be much of a burden, however. These are the two categories of seafood that tend to have the highest purine levels.

- Shellfish, such as shrimp and lobster, which— given their high price—are not staples of most diets; and

- Fish with dark meat, especially anchovies, herring, sardines, and mackerel, which are not among the most popular choices for most Americans

Milk and Other Dairy Products

In the next chapter, I will present a compelling case for including frequent servings of low-fat milk and other dairy products in your daily diet. Indeed, milk lives up to its wholesome image. Study after study has revealed that people who drink plenty of the white beverage and eat other dairy products weigh less than people who avoid these nourishing foods. One 2005 Iranian study, for instance, found that people who consume the most dairy foods cut their chances of becoming overweight or obese by up to 31 percent.

Dairy foods are an excellent source of calcium and vitamin D, and growing evidence suggests that the sugars and protein in milk and other dairy products lower uric acid levels in the blood, which will help you to control your weight and keep other health problems at bay. For example, a 2002 study published in the *Journal of the American Medical Association* showed that overweight young people who ate and drank frequent servings of dairy reduced their risk for developing full-blown metabolic syndrome by 72 percent.

WHAT'S TO DRINK?

Soda, fruit juice, and other beverages sweetened with sugar or high-fructose corn syrup are not permitted during the first 2 weeks of the Low-Fructose Diet and should be limited thereafter. You still have plenty of options, however. For starters, it's wise to follow the familiar advice about drinking plenty of water; 5 to 8 cups per day is a good goal. One easy way to achieve it is to keep a glass or bottle of water on hand at all times.

In terms of other beverages, drinking several glasses of low-fat milk every day may lower uric acid and have other important health benefits. And if you're a coffee lover, feel free to raise your mug: A 2007 study showed that people who drink a lot of the dark brew had lower uric acid levels—by 0.57 mg/dl, on average—than people who don't drink coffee. (You need a jitters-inducing 6 cups a day to get this benefit, however.)

You can also enjoy as much of the following beverages as you wish.

- Teas (unsweetened)

- Seltzer

- Diet soda and other artificially sweetened beverages (such as Crystal Light)

Fats and Oils

The critical message I want to deliver in this book is simple: Eating a high-fructose diet causes you to gain weight and develop other unhealthy conditions. Of course, it has never been my intention to suggest that fructose is the *only* danger lurking in the dietary landscape, of course. Fat matters, too. We eat too much of it, especially the unhealthy kinds. The Low-Fructose Diet limits your intake of bad fats, while encouraging you to include frequent servings of healthful fats that combine with other elements of the eating plan to combat metabolic syndrome.

There is no mystery to why eating a high-fat diet makes you gain weight. Fat provides 9 calories per gram—more than twice as many calories as protein and carbohydrates. There is little doubt: Eat too much dietary fat, and you will become fat.

. Of course, all fat is not created equal, and some types do far more harm than simply padding your hips and thighs. You know the main villain: saturated fat—found in juicy steaks, fried foods, ice cream, and butter—which raises LDL cholesterol, the kind that clogs arteries. It's just as important to avoid the trans fat in partially hydrogenated cooking oil, which is widely used by restaurants and food manufacturers (though many are bowing to public pressure and new legal restrictions, forcing them to use healthier alternatives). Trans fat raises the risk for heart disease, too. In fact, studies show that gram for gram, trans fat is the deadliest of all (see "Trans Fat: Bad for Your Belly and More," on the opposite page). Closely following the Low-Fructose Diet will help you to avoid both.

That said, the Low-Fructose Diet is not antifat. As you will see, I encourage you to enjoy delicious foods that are high in monounsaturated fat, such as avocados and nuts. Meanwhile, fish remains one of nature's best sources of omega-3 fatty acids, a superhealthy form of polyunsaturated fat. Omega-6 fatty acids are the other major "poly" in the American diet; the main sources are vegetable oils and margarine. Favoring monounsaturated and polyunsaturated fats over saturated and trans fats can improve your cholesterol levels and lower your risk for heart disease.

TRANS FAT:
BAD FOR YOUR BELLY AND MORE

A variety of processed foods, such as cookies, potato chips, and crackers, are prepared with partially hydrogenated oil. Many restaurants, especially fast-food eateries, rely on partially hydrogenated oil, too. The reason: Partially hydrogenated oil prolongs a food's shelf life and imparts other qualities that are difficult to achieve with butter or other oils.

Unfortunately, partially hydrogenated oil is full of trans fat. Trans fat has many downsides for your health. In fact, one study suggests that trans fat may cause unusually excessive weight gain, especially in the midsection—where extra pounds are the most dangerous.

A team of researchers at Wake Forest University School of Medicine fed diets containing about 35 percent fat, which is similar to the amount most Americans consume, to two groups of monkeys. For one group, about 8 percent of the calories came from trans fat, which would be typical of a person who consumes a great deal of fried food. For the other group, monounsaturated fat (primarily in the form of olive oil) replaced trans fat.

After 6 years, the body weight of the monkeys eating trans fat increased by 7.2 percent on average, compared with just 1.8 percent for the "control" monkeys. What's more, at the end of the study, the monkeys eating trans fat had 30 percent more abdominal fat. Abdominal fat is one of the five features of metabolic syndrome, and it increases the risk for heart disease and type 2 diabetes.

Though small amounts of trans fat occur naturally in meat and dairy products, processed foods are by far the main source of this fat in the American diet. Studies show that trans fat not only raises levels of LDL ("bad") cholesterol, it also reduces the size of LDL particles, making them more likely to clog arteries.

Furthermore, trans fat has much in common with fructose. Both elevate triglycerides, reduce HDL ("good") cholesterol, and trigger inflammation. Both fructose and trans fat increase the risk for heart disease and diabetes. Likewise, diets rich in trans fat have been linked to Alzheimer's disease.

The typical American consumes slightly less than 6 grams of trans fat every day, according to the USDA. The Low-Fructose Diet naturally lowers your intake, because many popular foods that are high in trans fat are also high in fructose, such as cookies, cakes, pies, and other baked snacks. Other common sources include margarine, french fries, potato chips, and corn chips. (Many of these products are now available without trans fats; check the Nutrition Facts label before you buy.)

Soft Drinks, Candy, and Desserts

These are the major sources of fructose in the American diet. In fact, 75 percent of the HFCS that we consume comes from this category alone. What's more, sweet foods and beverages account for 9 to 12 percent of the total calories that the average American consumes each day.

Nondiet soft drinks are the biggest culprits. A 12-ounce can of cola contains 20 grams of fructose, if not more; this is nearly an entire day's allowance. Fruit juice is another fructose powerhouse. Fruit "punch" and "cocktails"—which usually contain very little fruit—are often sweetened with large amounts of HFCS. (Beware: Some vegetable-based beverages may contain sugar, too.) Most sports drinks provide a modest dose of fructose.

While some critics have blamed soft drinks sweetened with HFCS for the obesity crisis, candy and desserts are major sources of fructose, too (whether in the form of refined sugar or HFCS). One of the worst offenders may be cake icing, which can deliver more than a day's worth of fructose—up to 50 grams—in ½ cup.

Normally, nutritionists suggest satisfying a sweet tooth with fresh fruit instead of candy and desserts. In order to limit your body's exposure to fructose during the first 2 weeks of my diet, fruit is off-limits during this period. For this reason, if you crave sweet-tasting beverages and snacks during this time, I recommend diet soft drinks and sugar-free freezer pops, candy, and baked goods. Despite some health concerns that have arisen about artificial sweeteners, I believe these products are reasonably safe and certainly a better choice than sugary drinks and snacks.

SIP, DON'T CHUG

Though reducing the *amount* of fructose in your diet is important, the *speed* at which you consume fructose matters, too. Studies show that uric acid levels soar much higher when fructose is ingested rapidly. This is a problem, because people often "chug" or guzzle soda and fruit juice, especially if they are hot or thirsty.

I remember one occasion when I was seated on a plane next to a young woman who ordered a cola from the flight attendant. I timed how long it took her to drink the entire 12-ounce can—just 3 minutes. Estimating her body weight, I did some quick calculations to determine that she had consumed the fructose in the cola fast enough to engage the metabolic pathway that produces uric acid.

This phenomenon may help to explain why beverages sweetened with sugar and high-fructose corn syrup are one of the driving forces behind the current epidemic of obesity in the United States and other countries. Soda may be particularly dangerous, because some studies suggest that carbonation accelerates the absorption of fructose.

The moral: If you simply cannot live without a sugar-sweetened soda, do yourself a favor—sip, don't chug.

Sugar Substitutes

If you have a sweet tooth, you may be concerned about feeling deprived when you adopt the Low-Fructose Diet. During the first 2 weeks, you will consume very little sugar. For some people, this will seem like a huge sacrifice, but it has a major, life-changing payoff: It will turn down the activity of fructose enzymes, which are responsible for all of the problems linked to fructose. As a result, you will lose weight and take control of the other metabolic problems I've described in this book. After the 2-week introductory phase of the diet, you can resume eating sugar, in small amounts.

The Low-Fructose Diet does allow for sugar-free foods and beverages, which get their sweet flavor from sugar substitutes. Because some controversy has surrounded these alternative sweeteners, you may be reluctant to use them. It's true that legitimate health concerns have been raised about the safety of consuming these products. Yet I believe that they offer a far safer alternative to foods and beverages sweetened with sugar, HFCS, and other sources of fructose.

Sugar substitutes are not for everyone for a simple reason: Some people don't like the way they taste, because food scientists have struggled to precisely match the qualities of sugar. But many find that the palate adapts over time, and they come to enjoy foods sweetened with sugar substitutes, which fall into two categories: artificial sweeteners and sugar alcohols.

For our purposes, it's essential to note one quality that products in both of these two groups share: None raise uric acid levels or produce any of the cellular damage that fructose can cause. Still, there are important differences between artificial sweeteners and sugar alcohols, which may influence your buying decisions as you read package labels. Let's take a closer look.

Artificial sweeteners

You know them by names such as Sweet'N Low and Equal, but scientists call these products "intense" or "nonnutritive" sweeteners. These descriptions sum up what's unique about artificial sweeteners: They are intensely sweet—hundreds of times sweeter than refined sugar. This means that you need only a tiny amount of an artificial sweetener to flavor a food or beverage. Artificial sweeteners provide no calories, or so few that they can be marketed as noncaloric. What's more, artificial sweeteners have no effect on blood sugar.

The FDA has approved five artificial sweeteners. Of the following list, you are probably most familiar with the first three, because they are commonly used as "tabletop" sweeteners (that is, replacements for table sugar), as well as food additives.

- Aspartame (NutraSweet and Equal), which is 200 times sweeter than sugar

- Saccharin (Sweet'N Low, Sweet Twin, and Necta Sweet), which is 200 to 700 times sweeter than sugar

- Sucralose (Splenda), which is 600 times sweeter than sugar

- Acesulfame-K (Sunett and Sweet One), which is 200 times sweeter than sugar

- Neotame, which is 7,000 to 13,000 times sweeter than sugar

Artificial sweeteners have been around for more than a century. The first, saccharin, was discovered in 1879. Controversy surrounding these faux sugars has been around for decades, too. For example, government scientists tried to ban saccharin in 1911, according to *FDA Consumer* magazine. Later, in the 1970s, studies of laboratory animals raised concerns that saccharin may cause bladder cancer. Subsequent investigations determined that moderate use of the sweetener (defined as less than six servings per day) is safe for humans. Major health organizations such as the American Cancer Society and American Dietetic Association approve of the use of saccharin.

Likewise, concerns have arisen about the safety of aspartame, which has been linked to an increased risk for brain cancer. But according to both the American Medical Association and the FDA, the weight of scientific evidence suggests that aspartame is safe. As a precaution, though, pregnant women should consume only moderate amounts of the sweetener.

At present, sucralose (better known as Splenda) is the most widely used artificial sweetener in the United States, accounting for nearly two-thirds of the market. Although the FDA allows Splenda to be promoted as providing no calories, it actually contains 2 calories per teaspoon. No serious health concerns have been linked to sucralose.

Here is the only major caveat about foods that contain artificial sweeteners: Avoid aspartame if you have a rare inherited condition called phenylketonuria. Aspartame partly converts to the amino acid phenylalanine in the body. People with phenylketonuria can't metabolize phenylalanine, so for them, aspartame can be toxic.

Sugar alcohols

Despite their somewhat misleading name, these sweeteners are not sugars and do not contain alcohol. Also known as polyols, these sugar substitutes are produced by altering the chemical structure of starch and other carbohydrates. (They also occur naturally in some fruits.) Food manufacturers use sugar alcohols in a variety of sugar-free foods, especially candy, cookies, and frozen desserts, as well as chewing gum.

Some of the more common varieties of sugar alcohol include maltitol, mannitol, sorbitol, and xylitol. The latter is as sweet as table sugar, while most other sugar alcohols are somewhat less sweet. Unlike sugar, polyols do not react with bacteria in the mouth, so they do not cause tooth decay. Nor do they elevate blood sugar.

Sugar alcohols differ from most artificial sweeteners in an important way: They are not calorie free. The typical sugar alcohol provides about 2 calories per gram. Although this is less than the 4 calories per gram in table sugar, you still need to keep portion control in mind when selecting foods sweetened with sugar alcohols. In other words, just because a product is labeled sugar free, eating too much can still cause weight gain, especially because the food may be high in fat, too.

A special problem exists with sorbitol and xylitol. Sorbitol breaks down into fructose, while xylitol behaves much like fructose once it is absorbed. The fact is, xylitol and sorbitol are generally not well absorbed by the body, but in some people up to 30 percent may reach the bloodstream. For this reason, foods containing sorbitol or xylitol could be another stealth source of fructose or its equivalent.

Also avoid any product that contains a form of sugar called tagatose (sometimes listed as D-tagatose), which may be combined with xylitol or other sugar substitutes. Although it is low in calories, tagatose is metabolized by fructose enzymes, so it will cause the same problems as fructose, such as stimulating production of uric acid.

One final reason to go easy on foods that contain sugar alcohols: In large doses, some polyols (especially mannitol and sorbitol) may cause bloating and diarrhea.

Salt

The Low-Fructose Diet is not a low-salt eating plan. Still, I encourage you to pay attention to how much salt you're consuming and to consider cutting back. Let me explain why.

Common salt is formed by two chemicals: sodium and chloride. Sodium is one of the body's major electrolytes, minerals in the blood that help to regulate many different biological processes. Sodium plays an important role in maintaining healthy blood volume. Eating too much salt can raise blood pressure, especially if you:

- Are over 60

- Are African American or

- Have diabetes

Furthermore, if you already have hypertension, consuming a salty diet can make it worse.

Even if you don't fit into any of these categories, however, your blood pressure may be creeping into the danger zone if you have been eating a high-fructose diet. In fact, we now know that people with the condition known as prehypertension (a systolic pressure between 120 and 139 and/or a diastolic pressure between 80 and 89) are at increased risk for heart disease.

Getting your salt intake under control can complement the other metabolic improvements you will experience as you reduce your body's exposure to fructose. Consider this: In a 2007 study, researchers gave instructions and advice on lowering salt intake to more than 1,100 people with prehypertension. Over a period of 10 to 15 years, these patients cut their heart attack risk by 25 percent, compared with a similar group of patients who did not restrict their salt intake.

The typical American consumes a great deal of salt—about 10 grams per day, or more than 2 teaspoons. I think it's wise to reduce that to no more than 5 or 6 grams, which is consistent with the positions of the federal government and organizations such as the American Heart Association.

Condiments, Spices, and Other Flavor Enhancers

There are many ways to add zest to a dish when you dine out or at home. Unfortunately, some of the most popular flavor boosters are stealth sources of fructose. Check the ingredients list on a bottle of ketchup, for instance, and you are bound to find HFCS or sugar. In fact, most brands of ketchup contain about 1.4 grams of fructose per serving, which can add up. Steak sauce, barbecue sauce, Worcestershire sauce, and many other toppings are high in sugar, too.

Another popular condiment, mustard, is usually fructose free (though there are exceptions, such as honey mustard). As always, the only way to know whether a condiment you purchase at the grocery store contains fructose is to read the label and look for sugar in its various forms.

To keep your calories under control and limit your intake of saturated fat, avoid full-fat versions of mayonnaise, tartar sauce, and salad dressings. On the other hand, feel free to make liberal use of nature's own flavoring agents, herbs and spices. Think of rosemary, cinnamon, oregano, garlic, and other natural seasonings as "free," because they provide few if any calories and have no effect on uric acid.

In fact, adding these plant-based flavor boosters to food may provide some health protection. A large analysis in the *American Journal of Clinical Nutrition* determined that herbs and spices are the food category with the highest concentration of antioxidants by weight.

Alcoholic Beverages

You can drink alcoholic beverages in moderation as part of the Low-Fructose Diet. But you will need to choose wisely. Some popular varieties can increase uric acid, while others actually help to control many of the metabolic problems created by a high-fructose diet.

Drinking alcohol stimulates production of uric acid. It also interferes with the kidneys' capacity to excrete uric acid. In theory, both of these effects can increase uric acid in the blood. In reality, though, the impact from alcohol itself—that is, ethanol, the common chemical in all alcoholic beverages—is pretty mild. It's the other ingredients in a drink that pose the bigger problem.

Unfortunately for lovers of ale and lager, beer contains large amounts of guanosine, a purine that converts to uric acid. Because of its high purine content, beer is probably the worst choice of all for people following the Low-Fructose Diet. Once again, we can say this based on what we know about gout patients, who have elevated uric acid. One study found that drinking just one beer per day increases the risk for gout by 50 percent.

As I mentioned in Chapter 5, beer's effect on uric acid may help to explain why people who drink excessive amounts of the popular malted beverage sometimes develop the dreaded "beer belly." Spirits seem to have a more modest overall effect, though cocktails made with fructose-rich soda pop or fruit juice could send uric acid soaring.

There is no scientific evidence that drinking wine raises uric acid (though sweet-tasting wines contain modest amounts of fructose). As you no doubt know, large population studies have revealed that people who consume small amounts of alcohol are actually healthier than teetotalers. It's no surprise that much of the early enthusiasm about the health benefits of alcohol focused on wine, thanks to the so-called French paradox. Cardiovascular disease is far less common in France than in the United States, despite the French affection for cheese and creamy sauces (to say nothing of cigarette smoking). Although the French eat less junk food and more fruits and vegetables than we do, they also drink more wine.

We know that small servings of wine, as well as other forms of alcohol, help to lower the risk for cardiovascular disease by raising levels of HDL cholesterol, the "good" kind. Moreover, wine—red wine, in particular—is brimming with an antioxidant known as resveratrol. (Peanuts and certain berries are good sources, too.) Resveratrol seems to protect the heart in a couple of ways. First, it prevents LDL cholesterol from becoming oxidized by free radicals, which in turn helps to keep arteries from narrowing. Second, studies of laboratory animals suggest that resveratrol may help to offset some of the ill effects of dietary fructose. Specifically, resveratrol increases production of nitric oxide and improves endothelial function, both of which are diminished when uric acid is too high. (Recent research suggests that white wine may offer substantial antioxidant protection, too.)

While one or two glasses of wine per day may have beneficial effects on cardiovascular health, exceeding this limit *increases* the risk for heart disease, high blood pressure, and liver damage—to say nothing of the psychological and social problems that accompany alcohol abuse. The benefits of drinking alcohol must always be balanced against the inherent risks.

CHAPTER 10

THE CASE FOR MILK

Dairy Foods and the
Low-Fructose Diet

"Got milk?" is one of the punchier advertising slogans in recent memory. Unfortunately, the answer from too many people today could be "Yes, but not much." The typical American drinks a little more than 21 gallons of milk each year. That's less than 1 cup per day and about half as much as Americans consumed after World War II. The steady decline in milk consumption in the United States occurred as sugar ascended and came to dominate our diets.

That's too bad, because milk and other dairy foods can help to counteract many of the problems I've described in this book, which arise when you overexpose your body to refined sugar and high-fructose corn syrup (HFCS). Think of milk as the antifructose, capable of speeding up weight loss, controlling blood pressure, and reducing heart disease risk. We're still learning how dairy foods keep you trim and safeguard your health, but growing evidence suggests that the sugar and protein in milk play important roles. What's

MILK: GOOD NEWS, BAD NEWS

The news about dairy consumption in the United States isn't all bad. Although Americans drank far more milk in the mid-1940s, it's important to note that most of it—41 gallons per year in 1945—was whole milk, which is high in artery-clogging saturated fat. Today, Americans drink less than 7 gallons of whole milk per year. Meanwhile, we consume roughly twice as much lower-fat milk today as we did a generation ago.

Unfortunately, one critical reason Americans aren't getting enough milk is that it's been displaced in our diets by sugar-sweetened soft drinks. A 2004 study by researchers at the University of North Carolina at Chapel Hill found that the number of calories coming from fructose-rich soda and fruit drinks shot up by 135 percent between 1977 and 2001. During the same period, consumption of milk, as measured in calories, dropped by 38 percent.

more, a diet rich in low-fat dairy foods confers an important advantage for fighting the effects of fructose: It lowers uric acid.

By now, most people are aware that dairy foods strengthen bones and help to prevent osteoporosis in both men and women. In recent years, however, low-fat milk and other dairy products have emerged as all-purpose nutritional saviors. Studies have shown that dairy lovers lose more weight more quickly than people who give up dairy products when they diet. Dairy foods have proven so effective at controlling hypertension that they help form the foundation of a widely used eating plan designed to lower blood pressure. Population studies suggest that dairy foods may help to cut the risk for type 2 diabetes, too.

Obviously, the essence of the Low-Fructose Diet is reducing your exposure to sugar, HFCS, and other sources of fructose. But adding certain foods to your diet is important, too. In the previous chapter, I discussed how each of the major food groups fits into my eating plan. Dairy is such an important counterweight to fructose that it deserves special attention.

Most adults consume about 1½ servings of milk and other dairy foods, on average, per day. If this describes you, then I believe you will experience marked health benefits simply by doubling your intake. Consider: When Harvard researchers analyzed the diets of more than 10,000 middle-aged women, they found that those who consumed at least three servings of dairy products per day cut their risk for developing metabolic syndrome by about one-third.

Dairy for Dieters

Because dairy foods are creamy and satisfying, many people stop eating them while trying to lose weight, believing that they *must* be fattening. It's a big mistake. Recent studies show that consuming low-fat dairy foods actually accelerates weight loss.

Dairy is the major source of calcium in the American diet. Between 70 and 75 percent of this mineral comes from milk and other dairy foods. We know from large population studies that people who consume a great deal of calcium tend to weigh less than their peers whose diets are low in this important mineral. We also know that low-calcium diets increase levels of hormones that prompt the body to store more fat and burn less.

Laboratory rats that are fed lots of dietary fat and sugar gain large amounts of body fat and burn less of it as energy if their diets contain little calcium. Adding calcium to a rat's diet has the opposite effect, causing the body to burn more fat and gain less.

So calcium is the key to dairy's weight-management magic, right? That's not clear. Several studies have shown that people lose more weight when they add a few daily servings of low-fat dairy foods to their diets than if they simply increase their calcium intake.

Nutritionist Michael Zemel, PhD, of the University of Tennessee, devised a study in which he placed obese people on one of three low-calorie diets. The first diet contained little dairy and calcium. The second was low in dairy but high in calcium, which came from mineral supplements. The third included plenty of dairy foods, delivering roughly the same amount of calcium as the second diet (1,200 to 1,300 milligrams per day).

After 6 months, the dairy group had the clear edge in weight loss, as you can see in the chart below.

DIET	WEIGHT LOSS AFTER 6 MONTHS (LB)
Low calcium, low dairy	14.5
High calcium, low dairy	18.9
High calcium, high dairy	24.4

Source: Obesity Research *12 (April 2004): 585.*

Dr. Zemel's study suggests that the calcium in dairy foods may have a more powerful effect on weight than calcium from dietary supplements. Or it could be that some other component of dairy foods promotes weight loss above and beyond any effect of calcium.

Dairy and Metabolic Syndrome: Early Clues

In 1982, long before pop stars and famous athletes began appearing in those ubiquitous "milk mustache" ads, researcher David McCarron, MD, discovered something surprising: High intake of dairy foods is associated with low blood pressure. Dr. McCarron, of Oregon Health Sciences University, and his colleagues analyzed the diets of 90 people—about half with essential hypertension, the most common form of high blood pressure, and the rest with healthy blood pressure. They found one striking difference in dietary habits between the two groups: Those with hypertension ate far fewer dairy foods than their counterparts with normal blood pressure.

Calcium plays a role in regulating blood pressure. To be sure, Dr. McCarron and his team found that the people with hypertension took in about 25 percent less calcium in their daily diets than those with normal blood pressure. On the other hand, there was no difference between the two groups in terms of their intakes of sodium and potassium, two electrolytes that help regulate blood pressure.

Larger studies have supported Dr. McCarron's finding that dairy foods, and calcium in particular, lower blood pressure. A government analysis of the diets of 10,000 American adults found that people who consume at least 1,000 milligrams of calcium per day cut their risk for high blood pressure by 40 to 50 percent. (The recommended intake of calcium for people age 19 and older is 1,000 milligrams per day; for men and women 51 and older, 1,200 milligrams per day.)

Inevitably, scientists posed the question: If calcium-rich dairy foods seem to lower blood pressure, why not treat hypertension with calcium supplements? Unfortunately, clinical trials have been inconsistent and disappointing. Some show a benefit, while others suggest that calcium pills do little to improve blood pressure.

In theory, increasing your calcium intake could actually *raise* blood pressure. Elevated levels of certain forms of calcium in vascular cells produce contractions, which cause blood vessels to constrict. High blood levels of calcium have been linked to hypertension in certain diseases, such as hyperparathyroidism.

While the idea of treating high blood pressure with calcium supplements never caught on, the case for consuming dairy foods has only gotten stronger. The National Institutes of Health sponsored the DASH (Dietary Approaches to Stop Hypertension) Study, a trial that compared a low-fat diet rich in fruits and vegetables with a similar diet that also included three servings of low-fat dairy foods daily. Because fruits and vegetables provide vitamin C and potassium, which play major roles in regulating blood pressure, it made sense that people in the first group saw a modest drop in blood pressure. As the chart below shows, eating several servings of dairy every day greatly enhanced this benefit.

	DROP IN SYSTOLIC BLOOD PRESSURE (MM HG)	DROP IN DIASTOLIC BLOOD PRESSURE (MM HG)
Low-fat diet rich in fruits and vegetables	7.2	2.8
Low-fat diet rich in fruits and vegetables *plus* 3 daily servings of low-fat dairy foods	11.4	5.5

Source: New England Journal of Medicine *336 (17 April 1997): 1120.*

This landmark 1997 study showed that combining low-fat dairy products with plenty of fruits and vegetables was about as effective as taking antihypertensive drugs. The authors of the DASH Study—which was published in the *New England Journal of Medicine*—estimated that if everyone who has hypertension ate more fruits, vegetables, and low-fat dairy foods, the number of heart attacks in the United States would drop by 15 percent, and strokes would decline by 27 percent.

To sum up, dairy foods have a consistent and powerful effect on blood pressure and weight, while calcium's benefits are questionable, at best. This suggests that milk, yogurt, and other dairy foods contain some other healthful compound. But what?

The Case for Vitamin D

The so-called "sunshine vitamin" provides at least part of the answer, because it seems to offset some of the ills associated with a high-fructose diet. Most milk sold in the United States is fortified with vitamin D, a program started in the 1930s to combat the childhood bone disease known as rickets. We know that vitamin D is essential to bone health over the life span, because it helps the body absorb calcium. According to growing evidence, this important vitamin also plays a critical role in preventing a variety of other diseases, including hypertension.

As its nickname suggests, vitamin D increases in the body when the skin is exposed to sunlight. This unusual phenomenon may help to explain a medical mystery that dates back to the early 1900s, when scientists observed that people who live in tropical lands near the equator tend to have very low blood pressure. By contrast, denizens of colder climates at higher latitudes have higher blood pressure.

Initially, scientists thought that temperature explained the geographic difference in blood pressure. Living in a hot climate makes you sweat more, so it was presumed that residents of the tropics lost more sodium in their per-spiration, which helped to keep their blood pressure low. Meanwhile, scientists theorized that cold weather activates the body's sympathetic nervous system, which governs our "fight or flight" response. Increased sympathetic nervous activity causes a number of biological changes—among them constricting blood vessels, which raises blood pressure.

These theories are interesting, but a better explanation seems to be that people who live in the tropics spend more time outdoors, exposed to the sun, so their skin synthesizes large amounts of vitamin D. Why does this matter? Recent research shows that vitamin D suppresses activity of the renin-angiotensin system (RAS), which produces hormones that regulate blood pressure. As activity of the RAS turns down, blood pressure drops.

What's more, population studies suggest that people with hypertension tend to have relatively low levels of vitamin D in their blood. According to animal studies, vitamin D can

---

DO YOU GET ENOUGH VITAMIN D?

Surveys indicate that many Americans are not getting enough vitamin D. The problem is especially acute among people over age 50.

Michael F. Holick, MD, of Boston University School of Medicine, and his colleagues reported that only 35 percent of Caucasian men and 6 women reached the recommended daily intake of vitamin D through diet and supplements; that figure drops to 17 percent among Latinos, and only 10 percent among African Americans. The latter statistic is especially troublesome, because skin pigment blocks ultraviolet light, making it harder for dark skin to produce vitamin D.

According to the National Academy of Science's Institute of Medicine, the adequate intake of vitamin D for people age 50 and younger is 200 IU per day; for people 51 to 70, 400 IU per day; and for people 71 and older, 600 IU per day. For reference, 1 cup of fortified milk provides 98 IU of vitamin D.

help protect against medical conditions linked to high blood pressure, including kidney disease and cardiac hypertrophy.

Gout Milk?

Another benefit of drinking milk is that it keeps uric acid under control. Doctors have known for centuries that frequent servings of milk can help limit flare-ups of gout, which is caused by high uric acid. The great 17th-century British philosopher John Locke recommended milk for gout, as did William Osler, MD, one of the fathers of modern medicine.

According to recent research, this was good advice. A large 2004 study published in the *New England Journal of Medicine (NEJM)* found that men who drank two glasses or more of fat-free milk every day were half as likely to develop gout as men who drank less than one glass per day. Low-fat yogurt offered similar protection.

We know that elevated uric acid not only causes gout, it also raises the risk for weight gain, high blood pressure, insulin resistance, and other problems. Further scientific evidence suggests that simply adding a serving or two of dairy products to your daily menu will help lower blood levels of uric acid.

The lead author of the *NEJM* paper, Massachusetts General Hospital rheumatologist Hyon K. Choi, MD, conducted another study that analyzed medical and nutrition data collected from nearly 15,000 Americans who had been interviewed as part of the third National Health and Nutrition Examination Survey between 1988 and 1994. Dr. Choi and his colleagues determined that consuming even modest amounts of dairy foods can make a big difference. For example, they found that uric acid levels are 0.25 mg/dl lower, on average, among people who drink just one glass of

A PROPHET-ABLE DRINK

One ancient Islamic medical text titled *Tibb-ul-Nabbi* (or *Medicine of the Prophet*) claimed that drinking milk "wipes away heat from the heart, strengthens the back, augments the intelligence, renews vision, and drives away forgetfulness," according to the *Journal of Dairy Science*.

milk or more each day, compared with people who never drink milk. Eating a serving of yogurt every other day had a similar beneficial effect on uric acid.

How Dairy Foods Lower Uric Acid

To understand how dairy foods lower uric acid, it helps to know a bit about a pair of organs you may not think about much: the kidneys. I happen to think about them a great deal, because my medical training is in nephrology, the branch of internal medicine that studies kidney function and disease.

The kidneys are two bean-shaped organs that sit at the rear of the abdomen, just above the waistline. As blood circulates through the kidneys, they filter out excess fluid and waste materials that are produced as part of normal metabolism, while returning precise amounts of salt, minerals, nutrients, and water to the blood supply. Excess fluid and waste products form urine, which passes out of the kidneys through slender tubes called ureters, into the bladder, and out of the body.

Most people do not realize that the kidneys have a wide variety of functions. They play a crucial role in regulating blood pressure, for example, and produce important hormones, including a form of vitamin D. As part of their filtering capacity, the kidneys perform another critical service: They take uric acid out of the blood and eliminate it through the urine. Research suggests that the kidneys perform this function more efficiently if you drink plenty of milk and consume other dairy products.

Milk helps lower uric acid levels for several reasons. For example, dairy foods contain a form of sugar known as lactose. During digestion, an enzyme called lactase breaks down lactose into simpler sugars, glucose and galactose. You may not be familiar with this latter sugar, but it appears to have a desirable influence on kidney function. Researchers at Mount Sinai Hospital in New York City produced evidence to suggest that galactose raises the amount of uric acid in the urine through its effects on special tubular cells in the kidneys. Increasing the volume of uric acid in the urine in turn lowers the concentration in the blood.

(By the way, some people produce too little lactase, so their bodies do not break down lactose. Lactase deficiency causes the condition known as lactose intolerance. Because they can't digest lactose, people with lactose intolerance can develop gastrointestinal problems if they consume dairy foods. But most people with lactose intolerance can enjoy at least some of the health benefits of milk and other dairy products; see "What If I'm Lactose Intolerant?")

Drinking milk and eating dairy foods such as yogurt seems to lower uric acid through at least one other mechanism, though we don't understand it quite as well. Along with galactose, milk protein appears to act on the kidneys to make them eliminate more uric acid.

A team of Canadian scientists demonstrated this in a study published in the *American Journal of Clinical Nutrition*. They asked 10 healthy volunteers to drink three different beverages on separate occasions. One solution contained water mixed with 80 grams of casein, the primary protein in milk; the second contained an equal amount of lactalbumin, another protein in milk; and the third contained soy protein. The researchers drew blood samples from the volunteers once an hour for 3 hours after drinking each beverage.

The soy milk caused the volunteers' uric acid levels to rise, probably because soy contains purines. On the other hand, uric acid dropped by about 0.5 mg/dl, on average, with the casein and lactalbumin beverage. This is an impressive reduction, though—to be fair—80 grams is a lot of milk protein. (By comparison, an 8-ounce glass of milk contains about 8 grams of protein.)

Still, this study offers clear evidence that drinking more low-fat milk and eating other dairy foods will help improve uric acid levels. We aren't sure exactly why this happens, though we have several theories. It could be, for example, that milk protein also interferes with how tubular cells process uric acid, causing more to be excreted in the urine.

Get Milk

If you were to scan a list of people who have posed for the National Milk Processor Board's "Got Milk?" ads, you couldn't help but notice that many are young, attractive, and trim. This is no coincidence. Adults tend to drink less and less milk as they reach middle age, so hinting that the white drink is a youthful elixir is one way to win back customers.

I can't promise that drinking more low-fat milk or eating yogurt and other dairy foods will make you look like pop singer Beyoncé Knowles or superstar quarterback Tom

---

WHAT IF I'M LACTOSE INTOLERANT?

Lactose intolerance affects about half of all adults worldwide but is particularly common among Asians, as well as Native Americans and African Americans. It occurs in people who lack the enzyme lactase, which breaks down lactose, the main sugar in milk. As undigested lactose enters the colon, gut bacteria feast on it, producing large amounts of hydrogen and other gases. As a result, consuming milk and other dairy products can lead to bloating, diarrhea, and other unpleasant gastrointestinal symptoms.

Most supermarkets carry milk and other dairy products that have been supplemented with lactase, which breaks down lactose into two simple sugars, glucose and galactose. In theory, people who are lactose intolerant can safely digest these sugars, though the reality is that they simply do not work for some people. If this is the case for you, you might experiment with milk, yogurt, and other dairy foods that are supplemented with live cultures, such as acidophilus and bifidum, which break down lactose.

You also might try portion control. A 2006 study in the *Journal of Nutrition* found that most people who are lactose intolerant can drink up to 1 cup of milk (preferably as part of a meal) without developing any symptoms.

Brady—just two of the many appealing celebrities to wear the famed milk mustache. But eating dairy foods will cancel out many of the effects of fructose, especially when you choose the rest of your diet carefully. I will show you how to do just that in the next chapter.

CHAPTER 11

THE LOW-FRUCTOSE DIET

Lose Weight and Beat Metabolic Syndrome the Low-Fructose Way

Until now, the title of this book may have seemed to be a comment on our collective obsession with sweet foods and beverages. All of us have heard a friend or colleague exclaim "I need my sugar fix!" as he or she eagerly unwraps a candy bar or slurps a bottle of soda. Maybe you have uttered those words from time to time.

The Sugar Fix has a second, more optimistic meaning. I believe it is possible to repair the damage done by a high-fructose diet and turn off the out-of-control biological mechanisms that are causing you to gain weight and increasing your risk for a number of serious diseases. Following the Low-Fructose Diet that I describe in the coming pages will give your body a fresh start—like rebooting a computer or changing the oil in your car.

The Low-Fructose Diet is designed to directly and aggressively attack the metabolic crisis caused by consuming excessive amounts of sugar, high-fructose corn syrup (HFCS), and other sources of fructose. This eating plan, which I developed with nutritionist and registered dietitian Elizabeth Gollub, PhD, is unique for several reasons.

The Low-Fructose Diet is based on science. Many popular diets sound logical, but when held to scientific scrutiny, they fail the test. Indeed, the diets featured in some best-selling books are completely lacking in scientific grounding. Some even promote unproven and potentially dangerous therapies, such as colonic enemas and herbal "fat burners."

The opposite is true of the Low-Fructose Diet. As the preceding pages make clear, a wealth of well-established science supports all of the recommendations I make in this chapter.

The Low-Fructose Diet targets the right carbohydrates. Low-carbohydrate diets have been the most popular weight-loss approach for years. The trouble is, they needlessly restrict some delicious foods that provide valuable health benefits. My eating plan targets the carbohydrate you need to avoid—fructose—so you can enjoy others that will not make you fat or sick.

The Low-Fructose Diet lowers uric acid. Unlike any other diet you may have tried, the eating plan I'm about to describe is designed to reduce blood levels of uric acid by minimizing your body's exposure to fructose and purines. Other diets may produce a modest drop in uric acid, but none is structured to induce a significant drop in this critical compound.

The Low-Fructose Diet corrects your level of fructose enzymes. If you are overweight or you have conditions of metabolic syndrome, then your fructose enzymes are likely too high. The Low-Fructose Diet addresses this problem by reducing the volume and activity of these all-important enzymes. Low-carb diets may produce the same effect, but to a lesser degree.

People who have adopted the Low-Fructose Diet say that it has helped them learn how to make better food choices, so they could lose any extra pounds and maintain a healthy weight. Avoiding sweets became natural. Furthermore, because they had lowered their fructose enzymes, their bodies were better able to accommodate an occasional candy bar or slice of birthday cake. Many say that they were able to enjoy life more, because they no longer worried about how to lose weight or keep it off.

How the Diet Works

The Low-Fructose Diet is really two diets in one, because it allows you to choose between a pair of distinct approaches to weight loss. You simply select the option that suits you better.

Both versions of the diet have the same basic structure. Each consists of an initial 2-week phase during which you must reduce your fructose intake to a bare minimum. I will show you how to eliminate as much fructose from your daily menu as possible. After this 14-day phase, you will reintroduce fructose to your diet, though moderation is the key: The low-fructose lifestyle I recommend includes one-third to one-half the amount of fructose currently consumed by most Americans.

The only difference between the two versions of the Low-Fructose Diet is how you choose to undertake the first phase. Option One is the simpler of the two. It does not require you to count calories or do any other tabulating. You simply select the foods you wish to eat from a list I'll provide. Option One is best for:

- People who have a history of eating and drinking a large amount of fructose-rich foods and beverages and

- People who have metabolic syndrome, with at least three of the following five conditions: obesity (especially in the midsection), high blood pressure, elevated triglycerides, low HDL cholesterol, and elevated blood glucose

Option Two is more structured and specific. It requires you not only to avoid fructose but also to count calories. The obvious advantage of choosing Option Two is that you will probably lose more weight more quickly. But it also requires a bit more planning and commitment. I believe that Option Two is best for:

- People who have a serious weight problem— that is, a body mass index (BMI) of 30 or higher (see page 105 to determine your BMI)

- People who have failed on several other weight-loss diets and

- People who prefer a formal, detailed eating plan

Choose the version of my diet that best matches your needs. Option One is less restrictive and easier to follow, while Option Two may produce faster results. You will lose weight and improve your all-around health with either option.

Although both options require you to avoid foods that contain fructose during the initial 2 weeks, most people handle this stage without much trouble. After all, consuming large amounts of fructose every day is *not* natural for humans, so it's not as if I were asking you to change your diet in a way that will feel foreign or strange. This isn't always the case with weight-loss diets, because some drastically limit entire categories of macronutrients, such as fat or carbohydrates. While you may lose weight on one of these extreme diets, they are notoriously difficult to maintain. The reason: They require you to eat in an unnatural way.

The Low-Fructose Diet is not an extreme eating plan. In fact, even the low-calorie option I offer breaks down as 50 to 55 percent carbohydrates, 25 to 30 percent fat, and 20 percent protein. Humans have been eating a similar macronutrient composition for centuries, so most people will find it familiar and quite acceptable.

Sweet Liberation: The Fructose-Free Phase

No matter which version of the Low-Fructose Diet you choose, to begin the diet you must dramatically limit your fructose intake for 2 weeks. I call this 14-day period the Fructose-Free Phase. It is the most important aspect of the diet. The goal and purpose is straightforward: Keep as much fructose as possible out of your system for 2 weeks.

By removing fructose from your diet for this brief period, you will reduce the levels of fructose enzymes in your cells and rein in their out-of-control activity. Fructose enzymes are responsible for all of fructose's ill effects. If you are overweight or have other conditions of metabolic syn-

IF YOU HAVE DIABETES

The Low-Fructose Diet is designed for people who are overweight and have conditions of metabolic syndrome—among them insulin resistance, which precedes type 2 diabetes. If you have already been diagnosed with type 2 diabetes, the Low-Fructose Diet can still help you control your weight, blood pressure, blood fats, and other symptoms, though you will need to make some adjustments.

Some foods that are low in fructose have a relatively high glycemic index. That is, they cause blood glucose levels to rise rapidly—just what people with diabetes need to avoid. For this reason, you may need to limit your intake of starchy foods such as potatoes and rice. Furthermore, if you have diabetes, you may need to adjust what you eat based on what medications you're taking or how physically active you are on a given day.

As always, your best bet is to talk to your doctor, diabetes educator, or registered dietitian about a diet that is appropriate for you.

---

drome, then your fructose enzymes very likely are too high, and they have become overactive. In this case, eating even small servings of fructose will slow down weight loss and trigger all of the unhealthy metabolic changes I've described in the preceding chapters.

Studies show that giving your body a break from fructose causes the levels of fructose enzymes in your cells to drop. Once you have corrected this problem, you can resume eating small servings of foods that contain sugar, because exposure to a limited amount of fructose will no longer set off the chain of events that prompts fat cells to fill up, become inflamed and insulin resistant, and produce excessive amounts of uric acid, leading to other metabolic problems.

The result? Shedding pounds and maintaining a healthy weight will become much easier. Furthermore, as you lower your uric acid and block the unhealthy metabolic pathways activated by fructose, your health will improve and you will gain important protection against high blood pressure, type 2 diabetes, kidney disease, and other potentially devastating conditions.

Although I call the introductory period the Fructose-Free Phase, you will still be consuming very small amounts of fructose, because it is neither feasible nor wise to eliminate all foods that contain sugar outside of a controlled laboratory setting. After all, some very healthful foods—such as vegetables—contain small amounts of fructose.

The Fructose-Free Phase: Option One

Option One could not be simpler: Choose foods from the lists that I will provide, and avoid certain other foods. It's that easy. There is no need to count calories, carbs, or fat grams. Instead, use the lists to decide what to eat every day. If an item is not on the list, don't eat it.

The major difference between the foods you can and cannot eat during the Fructose-Free Phase is, of course, their fructose content. All of the foods that you are allowed to eat during this 2-week period contain less than 1 gram of fructose in a standard serving. In fact, the majority have less than 0.5 gram per serving. Eating only foods on this list and avoiding all others will lower your levels of fructose enzymes.

As you will see, limiting your diet to foods that contain no more than 1 gram of fructose per serving rules out many common foods, yet allows a long list of other favorites. For example, while I'm asking you to forgo carrots and peas for 2 weeks, you can still have asparagus and spinach with your dinner.

Some of the limitations may surprise you. For instance,

CASE STUDY: LOSING "LOVE HANDLES"

Michael Jessup underwent a kidney and pancreas transplant in 1999, which essentially cured him of type 1 diabetes, a disease he had lived with for 28 years. As a result, Michael was free to indulge in forbidden foods, such as chocolate. But splurging on sweets, along with taking medication he needed after his surgery, had a downside: Michael gained 40 pounds. "I had a basketball gut," says Michael, who lives in Baltimore, Maryland, with his wife and two children.

Michael tried several popular weight-loss diets, but none worked. I advised him to eliminate as much fructose as possible and to cut back on foods rich in purines. Six weeks later, Michael had lost 14 pounds and planned to shed 20 more. "The love handles are gone," he said, and his "basketball gut" was rapidly deflating.

Cutting out sweets and giving up his beloved shrimp (which are rather high in purines) wasn't easy at first, says Michael, but he quickly adjusted. He now searches for fructose in the ingredient lists of product labels when shopping for groceries, which has helped change his perspective on food. "The nicest thing about going on this diet is that I have become very conscious about what I eat," says Michael. "I feel great."

you may wonder: Isn't whole grain bread healthier than sourdough bread? It may be, in some respects. But many common brands of whole grain and whole wheat bread contain a substantial amount of added sugar or HFCS. Unless you are certain that a loaf was baked without added sweeteners, avoid it.

Among its many benefits, eliminating fructose from your diet will help bring down your uric acid. To reduce it even further, I'll show you how to avoid foods that are high in purines during the Fructose-Free Phase and beyond.

Foods to choose during the Fructose-Free Phase

The foods in the following lists either are free of fructose or contain less than 1 gram of fructose per serving. During the Fructose-Free Phase, eat only foods from these lists.

Vegetables

Alfalfa sprouts

Artichokes

Asparagus

Avocados (technically
a fruit)

Brussels sprouts

Cabbage (green)

Cauliflower

Celery

Collards

Endive

Garlic

Green beans

Kale

Leeks

Lettuce (all varieties)

Mushrooms

Mustard greens

Okra

Olives (technically
a fruit)

Parsley

Pickles, dill

Potatoes (russet only)

Radishes

Rhubarb

Sauerkraut

Spinach

Squash, yellow

Swiss chard

Tomatoes [1]

Turnip greens

Watercress

Yams [2]

Breads and Pasta

Biscuits, plain or
buttermilk

English muffin
(sourdough)

Matzo, plain

Melba toast

Pasta (all varieties)

Pita, white

[1] Tomatoes are somewhat high in fructose, so limit yourself to one half per day.

[2] Don't confuse yams with sweet potatoes; the latter have a rather high fructose content.

Pumpernickel bread

Rye bread

Sourdough bread

Tortillas, corn or flour

Grains

Barley

Bulgur

Rice, white or brown

Wild rice

Meat and Poultry

Beef

Chicken

Lamb

Pork

Turkey

Fish

Albacore tuna

Halibut

Lake trout

Salmon

Sole

Other white- or lighter-fleshed varieties

Breakfast Cereals

Cheerios (toasted whole grain oat variety only)

Cream of Wheat

Grape-Nuts

Grits

Oatmeal

Shredded wheat

Legumes

Adzuki beans

Black beans

Chickpeas or garbanzo beans

Cowpeas or black-eyed peas

Lentils

Soybeans (tofu)

Nuts and Seeds

Almonds

Brazil nuts

Hazelnuts or filberts

Macadamia nuts

Peanuts

Pecans

Pumpkin seeds

Sesame seeds

Sunflower seeds

Walnuts

Condiments

Garlic

Lemon juice

Mustard (except honey mustard)

Salsa

Sugar-free salad dressing

Tabasco sauce

Vinegar

Dairy

Cheese (low-fat varieties are preferable)

Milk (low fat or fat free is preferable)

Yogurt, plain (unflavored)

Fats and Oils

No specific limitations; olive and canola oils are the best choices

Dessert and Snack Foods

Club crackers

Popcorn

Pretzels

Ritz crackers

Saltines

Sugar-free cookies, cakes, and frozen treats

Triscuits

Beverages

Coffee (unsweetened)

Diet soda and other sugar-free beverages

Seltzer

Teas (unsweetened)

Off the menu: foods to avoid

The following foods are high in fructose and purines. Eating them during the Fructose-Free Phase will interfere with the goal of lowering fructose enzymes and uric acid. Do not consume any of the foods mentioned below for the first 2 weeks of the diet.

High-Fructose Foods

During the Fructose-Free Phase, you should avoid any food or beverage that contains significant amounts of naturally occurring or added fructose. The most obvious items on the list include:

Candy	Honey
Cookies, cakes, pies, and other baked goods	Soda and other soft drinks (other than diet varieties)
Fruit	
Fruit juice and other beverages that contain fruit (such as fruit punch)	Sports drinks

These are only the most obvious sources of fructose. Beware in particular when purchasing processed foods, because many contain added sugar and HFCS.

Unless you prepare every meal you eat from scratch, avoiding fructose requires some sleuthing in the form of carefully examining labels on packaged foods or asking restaurant servers whether a menu item contains added sugar. Unfortunately, sugar goes by many different names and comes in a variety of forms.

Most of the terms below are simply variations of sucrose, or table sugar. Do not eat any products that mention these stealth sources of fructose on their labels:

Beet sugar	Corn sweetener
Brown sugar	Corn syrup*
Cane sugar	Demerara sugar

*Most corn syrup products consist primarily of glucose (also known as dextrose), which has no effect on the mechanisms I have described in this book that cause obesity. Still, be sure to read package labels, because some products labeled as "corn syrup" are actually a blend of glucose and fructose.

Fruit juice concentrate

Granulated sugar

High-fructose corn
syrup

Honey

Invert sugar

Maple syrup

Molasses

Muscovado sugar

Raw sugar

Sucrose

Syrup

Table sugar

Tagatose

Turbinado sugar

High-Purine Foods and Beverages

Avoiding high-purine foods and beverages (including beer, which is very high in purines) during the Fructose-Free Phase will help drive down your uric acid levels. After the Fructose-Free Phase, you can include limited amounts of high-purine foods in your diet. (See "The Purine Content of Selected Foods" on page 370.)

Tips for getting the most from Option One

Eliminating fruit from your diet for 2 weeks means you may be missing some important nutrients. For this reason, I recommend taking the following dietary supplements every day.

- A multivitamin/mineral, which will ensure that you're getting the recommended daily amounts of essential nutrients

- 250 milligrams of vitamin C, which will provide additional antioxidant protection and may help lower uric acid

After completing the Fructose-Free Phase, you may want to continue taking a daily multivitamin/mineral supplement and a vitamin C supplement (especially the latter; I'll explain why in the next chapter). Here are a few additional strategies to help you successfully navigate the Fructose-Free Phase.

- Not all foods come in packages with adequate nutrition information. During this 2-week period, avoid any packaged product that does not provide an ingredient list.

- Consider avoiding restaurants and takeout food while you're on the Fructose-Free Phase unless you know for certain that the meals you want to order do not contain sugar or HFCS.

- If you would like to sweeten any food, such as breakfast cereal or coffee, use an artificial sweetener such as aspartame (NutraSweet and Equal), saccharin (Sweet'N Low and others), or sucralose (Splenda).

- Try to drink 5 to 8 cups of water per day (that is, in addition to any sugar-free beverages you may consume).

- You may drink alcoholic beverages in moderation during the Fructose-Free Phase, but only dry wine and spirits—no beer. Limit yourself to two drinks per day. A glass of wine equals 5 ounces; a shot of vodka, gin, or other spirit is $1^1/2$ ounces. Do not drink cocktails made with fruit juice, nondiet soda, or any other mixer that contains sugar or HFCS.

The Fructose-Free Phase: Option Two

If you choose to follow Option One of the Fructose-Free Phase, you can expect to lose weight, especially if you have been in the habit of consuming a lot of foods that contain sugar and HFCS. Option Two achieves the same primary goal as Option One—it lowers your levels of fructose enzymes—but it also is a traditional weight-loss diet, because you will limit your daily calories. For this reason, most people will lose weight more quickly with Option Two.

In exchange for speedier weight loss, you will need to do a little more work. Once again, how much is up to you. Here's what I mean: I am going to offer three different daily calorie intakes for you to choose from, depending on your gender, activity level, and personal preferences. While maintaining your daily calorie intake, you must

---

CASE STUDY: THE PROBLEM WITH FRUIT

Rita Bernuy, 34, was frustrated; her weight had reached 165 pounds. So she gave up sugary foods and started exercising regularly. Within 1 month, she lost 7 pounds. Then she hit a plateau. Her weight wouldn't budge.

When Rita and I talked about her diet, I discovered that that she was eating five or six servings of fruit every day—mostly fresh-squeezed orange juice, apples, and bananas. I advised her to continue avoiding foods that contained added sugar, but also to stop eating fruit for 2 weeks.

After 1 week, Rita lost 5 pounds. After 2 weeks, I told her she could have one serving of fruit per day. Over the next month, she continued to lose weight, ultimately dropping an additional 20 pounds. She has maintained this weight loss by continuing to eat a low-fructose diet.

choose foods that are low in fructose and low in purines. In addition, you will need to watch your portion sizes in order to keep a tight rein on calories.

How? You could select foods from the lists starting on page 350 and use a calorie-counting guide to help you decide how much you can eat. (Calorie-counting guides are available at supermarkets and bookstores; some Web sites provide the same information.) Counting calories yourself and measuring portion sizes is not difficult, but it does take some time and planning.

On the other hand, you could let us do the work for you. Starting on page 219, you will find 14 different daily menus that I call Day Plans. Each Day Plan features a different lineup of meals, but always a breakfast, lunch, dinner, and two snacks. Further, each Day Plan has been configured to provide the same healthy balance of protein, carbohydrates, fat,

---

FRUCTOSE WITHDRAWAL?

If you are accustomed to eating a lot of sugary foods, you may develop some unpleasant symptoms during the Fructose-Free Phase. They can be as mild as a craving or desire to eat sweets. In rare cases, though, people develop symptoms similar to those experienced by coffee drinkers who go through caffeine withdrawal after giving up their daily brew, such as headaches and fatigue.

It's not clear whether this phenomenon occurs because your body suddenly feels deprived of fructose or simply because you are eating less food, so you have less fuel to burn. Regardless, a few steps may help.

First, a craving for sweets may actually be a sign of dehydration, so be sure to drink plenty of water—5 to 8 cups a day is a good goal. If cravings for sweets persist, you might try having a small serving of sugar-free chocolate or a sugar-free baked good. (If you choose the low-calorie version of the Fructose-Free Phase, keep in mind that you may have only two snacks per day.) Most important, know that these symptoms tend to fade quickly and disappear altogether once you move on to the next phase of the diet.

> ## CASE STUDY: FRUCTOSE FREEDOM
> ## RELIEVES METABOLIC SYNDROME
>
> Ken, 46, was moderately overweight at 205 pounds. He also had mild hypertension and elevated triglycerides—a classic case of metabolic syndrome. Clearly, his diet was a problem, because he ate candy and drank soda and sweetened iced tea every day.
>
> Once Ken cut back on all foods containing fructose, he lost 15 pounds, and his blood pressure dropped from 140/92 to 120/70—an impressive reduction. Furthermore, his fasting triglycerides fell from 230 mg/dl to 70 mg/dl, greatly reducing his risk for heart disease. Tests showed that his kidney function had improved, too.

and fiber, while precisely controlling your calories and dramatically limiting the amount of fructose you will consume.

Very important: You needn't follow each one of the 14-Day Plans. Doing so would require you to buy quite a lot of food. Instead, choose Day Plans that appeal to you and stick with them. This will allow you to shop economically and won't force you to eat foods that don't interest you. Of course, if you like a lot of variety and enjoy trying new dishes, feel free to follow as many of the 14-Day Plans as you wish. You will probably find it easier to select a handful that work for you and make them the foundation of your 2-week Fructose-Free Phase.

One last thing: Please don't mix and match meals from one Day Plan to the next. Each Day Plan has been carefully designed to provide the necessary balance of nutrients and calories while dramatically limiting your fructose intake.

Choose your calories

Calorie needs vary from one person to the next, depending on gender and activity level. We've accounted for these differences by creating three different versions of Option Two.

- The 1,200-calorie version is best for women who want rapid, substantial weight loss.

- The 1,600-calorie version is for men who want rapid, substantial weight loss. It's also a good choice for active women who exercise regularly.

- The 2,000-calorie version is for active men who exercise regularly.

Think of your daily calorie total as a guide, not an iron-clad rule. When you reduce the number of calories you consume every day, it's not unusual to feel hungry now and then, especially at first. If constant hunger becomes a distraction, feel free to eat slightly larger portions of food than the menu recommends, or switch to a higher calorie intake. You will lose weight during the Fructose-Free Phase as long

---

ARE YOU READY? ARE YOU SURE?

You may think that losing weight and keeping it off requires the special and ineffable quality called willpower. But psychologists say that another emotional factor predicts diet success: readiness to change behaviors. They have shown that people who embark on diets are far more likely to lose weight and keep it off if they've made a complete emotional commitment to altering their eating patterns. For example, you must be willing to:

- Spend the necessary time to plan and prepare healthy meals

- Make sacrifices, such as cutting back on or giving up favorite foods, or temporarily altering your social schedule to avoid circumstances where you will be tempted to overeat

- Tolerate a growling belly now and then during the most-restrictive periods of a diet

In short, you need to be mentally willing to give up a few things in exchange for a slimmer waistline and better health.

as you avoid foods containing 1 gram of fructose or more. The Low-Fructose Diet will also reduce your fructose enzymes, which will help you avoid weight gain in the future.

Whether you decide to count calories on your own or follow the Day Plans, take a daily multivitamin/mineral supplement to ensure that you are getting the recommended levels of essential nutrients, just as with Option One. Also, take 250 milligrams of vitamin C, which will provide additional antioxidant protection and may help lower uric acid.

Day Plans for Option Two

The charts that follow present 14 daily menus to select from if you choose Option Two of the Fructose-Free Phase. Pick any Day Plan that appeals to you—though as a reminder, do not mix and match meals from one day to another. The left-hand column displays a given day's entire menu. The next three columns represent the different calorie intakes. Scan down the appropriate column for the calorie-controlled plan you have selected to determine portion sizes. Note: There are slight differences in the foods included in each plan, so any foods that are not part of a meal for your plan are noted with a "—" mark.

Each Day Plan specifies the basic foods allowed. Use these guidelines when cooking.

- Do not add sugar, honey, or any other source of fructose to a dish.

- Salt is acceptable, but it should be kept to a minimum.

- You can use most herbs and spices liberally.
  Check the labels of specially packaged
  preparations to make sure they don't contain
  sugar.

- You can use the following amounts of
  condiments to flavor your meals every day.
    1 tablespoon yellow, brown, or horseradish mustard
    2 tablespoons vinegar (check labels; some contain
      added sugar)
    1 tablespoon lemon juice
    1 teaspoon Tabasco sauce
    2 tablespoons soy or tamari sauce (check labels;
      some contain added sugar)

- For cooking oil, use canola or olive oil. The
  following amounts are permitted per day.
    1,200-calorie plan—1 teaspoon
    1,600-calorie plan—2 teaspoons
    2,000-calorie plan—1 tablespoon

DAY 1

	1,200 CALORIES	1,600 CALORIES	2,000 CALORIES
Breakfast			
Sourdough English muffin, toasted	1	1	1
Swiss cheese	1-ounce slice	1-ounce slice	1-ounce slice
Hot oatmeal	—	—	¾ cup
Sugar-free breakfast syrup	—	—	1 ounce
Lunch			
Chicken noodle soup	1 cup	1½ cups	1½ cups
Fresh celery	2 ribs	2 ribs	2 ribs
Ranch salad dressing, fat free	2 tablespoons	2 tablespoons	2 tablespoons
Pumpernickel roll	1 medium	1 medium	—
Rye bread	—	—	2 slices
Soft-spread margarine	—	—	2 teaspoons
Afternoon snack			
Low-fat frozen yogurt, sugar free (nonfruit flavor)	½ cup	½ cup	1 cup
Dinner			
Roasted skinless chicken breast topped with 2 chopped garlic cloves, sautéed in 1 tablespoon olive oil	3 ounces	4 ounces	5 ounces
White long-grain rice	½ cup	¾ cup	1 cup
Steamed asparagus	5 spears	5 spears	5 spears
Evening snack			
Rold Gold Tiny Twists fat-free pretzels	18 pretzels	25 pretzels	30 pretzels

DAY 2

	1,200 CALORIES	1,600 CALORIES	2,000 CALORIES
Breakfast			
Cheerios	1 cup	1½ cups	2 cups
Low-fat milk	¾ cup	¾ cup	1 cup
Rye bread, toasted	1 slice	1 slice	1 slice
Soft-spread margarine	1 teaspoon	1 teaspoon	1 teaspoon
Lunch			
Pita, white (fill with next three items to make a sandwich)	1 medium (about 6 inches in diameter)	1 medium (about 6 inches in diameter)	1 large (about 8 inches in diameter)
Sesame tahini	2 tablespoons	2 tablespoons	3 tablespoons
Alfalfa sprouts	1 cup	1 cup	1 cup
Sliced mushrooms	½ cup	½ cup	½ cup
Afternoon snack			
Fudgsicle ice cream bar, sugar free	1	1	—
Low-fat frozen yogurt, sugar free (nonfruit flavor)	—	—	1 cup
Dinner			
Broiled salmon fillet	4 ounces	5 ounces	6 ounces
Wild rice	½ cup	1 cup	1½ cups
Steamed yellow squash	½ cup	½ cup	½ cup
Ranch salad dressing, fat free (for squash)	—	—	1 tablespoon
Evening snack			
Low-fat microwave popcorn	3 cups	3 cups	3 cups
Low-fat hot cocoa, sugar free	—	1 cup	1 cup

DAY 3

	1,200 CALORIES	1,600 CALORIES	2,000 CALORIES
Breakfast			
Cream of Wheat	1 cup	1 cup	1½ cups
Sugar-free breakfast syrup	2 ounces	2 ounces	2 ounces
Chopped walnuts	1 tablespoon	2 tablespoons	¼ cup
Lunch			
Roasted turkey (for sandwich)	3 ounces	3 ounces	3 ounces
Sourdough bread	2 slices	2 slices	2 slices
Baked potato chips	11 chips	15 chips	20 chips
Afternoon snack			
Low-fat frozen yogurt, sugar free (nonfruit flavor)	½ cup	¾ cup	1 cup
Dinner			
Black beans	½ cup	1 cup	1½ cups
White rice	½ cup	1 cup	1½ cups
Fresh mixed salad greens	2 cups	2 cups	2 cups
Light Italian salad dressing, sugar free	2 tablespoons	2 tablespoons	2 tablespoons
Evening snack			
Reduced-fat Triscuits	7 crackers	10 crackers	10 crackers
Extra-sharp Cheddar cheese	—	—	1 ounce

DAY 4

	1,200 CALORIES	1,600 CALORIES	2,000 CALORIES
Breakfast			
Grape-Nuts	½ cup	½ cup	¾ cup
Low-fat milk	¾ cup	¾ cup	1 cup
Lunch			
Macaroni or other pasta	1 cup	1½ cups	1½ cups
Melted low-fat cheese, shredded (to make macaroni and cheese)	¼ cup	⅓ cup	⅓ cup
Fresh celery	2 ribs	2 ribs	2 ribs
Radishes	5	5	5
Light Italian salad dressing, sugar free (for dipping vegetables)	—	1 tablespoon	2 tablespoons
Afternoon snack			
Chocolate-vanilla swirl pudding cup, sugar free	1 snack cup	1 snack cup	1 snack cup
Dinner			
Grilled sirloin steak or skinless chicken breast	3 ounces	4 ounces	5 ounces
Rice pilaf	½ cup	1 cup	1½ cups
Steamed green beans	½ cup	½ cup	½ cup
Light Italian salad dressing, sugar free (for beans)	1 tablespoon	2 tablespoons	Instead of salad dressing, top snap beans with 2 chopped garlic cloves sautéed in 1 tablespoon of olive oil
Evening snack			
Rold Gold Tiny Twists fat-free pretzels	18 pretzels	18 pretzels	25 pretzels
Low-fat hot cocoa, sugar free	—	1 cup	1 cup

DAY 5

	1,200 CALORIES	1,600 CALORIES	2,000 CALORIES
Breakfast			
Poached egg	1 large	1 large	1 large
Sourdough English muffin, toasted	1	1	1
Soft-spread margarine	1 teaspoon	1 teaspoon	2 teaspoons
Lunch			
Chicken barley soup	1 cup	1½ cups	2 cups
Low-fat whole wheat crackers	7 crackers	10 crackers	10 crackers
Jalapeño jack soy cheese	2 slices	2 slices	2 slices
Afternoon snack			
Fudgsicle ice cream bar, sugar free	1	1	Have a sugar-free pudding cup instead
Chopped walnuts	—	2 tablespoons	2 tablespoons
Dinner			
Roasted turkey	3 ounces	4 ounces	5 ounces
Mashed russet potatoes	½ cup	½ cup	1 cup
Steamed spinach	½ cup	½ cup	½ cup
Turkey gravy, fat free	¼ cup	⅓ cup	⅓ cup
Evening snack			
Low-fat microwave popcorn	3 cups	3 cups	Instead of popcorn, have 2 slices of rye bread with 2 tablespoons low-fat cream cheese, with 1 cup low-fat, sugar-free hot cocoa

DAY 6

	1,200 CALORIES	1,600 CALORIES	2,000 CALORIES
Breakfast			
Hot oatmeal	1 cup	1½ cups	1½ cups
Low-fat hot cocoa, sugar free	1 cup	1 cup	—
Chopped walnuts	—	—	¼ cup
Lunch			
Tuna, water packed (for sandwich with next three items)	½ cup	¾ cup	1 cup
Rye bread	2 slices	2 slices	2 slices
Light mayonnaise	1 teaspoon	2 teaspoons	1 tablespoon
Alfalfa sprouts	½ cup	½ cup	1 cup
Baked potato chips	—	20 chips	20 chips
Afternoon snack			
Low-fat frozen yogurt, sugar free (nonfruit flavor)	½ cup	½ cup	1 cup
Rold Gold Tiny Twists fat-free pretzels	—	18 pretzels	20 pretzels
Dinner			
Spinach pasta	1 cup	1½ cups	1½ cups
Light Alfredo sauce (for pasta)	¼ cup	¼ cup	⅓ cup
Fresh mixed salad greens	1 cup	1 cup	2 cups
Creamy French salad dressing, sugar free	1 tablespoon	1 tablespoon	2 tablespoons
Evening snack			
Roasted salted soy nuts	¼ cup	⅓ cup	½ cup

DAY 7

	1,200 CALORIES	1,600 CALORIES	2,000 CALORIES
Breakfast			
Egg substitute	½ cup	1 cup	1 cup
Low-fat shredded Cheddar cheese	2 tablespoons	2 tablespoons	⅓ cup
Sourdough English muffin, toasted	1	1	1
Soft-spread margarine	1 teaspoon	1 teaspoon	2 teaspoons
Lunch			
Pita bread (fill with next two items to make sandwich)	1, about 4-inch diameter	1, about 6½-inch diameter	2, about 6½-inch diameter
Hummus spread	4 tablespoons	4 tablespoons	4 tablespoons
Alfalfa sprouts	½ cup	½ cup	1 cup
Rold Gold Tiny Twists fat-free pretzels	18 pretzels	18 pretzels	20 pretzels
Afternoon snack			
Chocolate-vanilla swirl pudding cup, sugar free	1	1	Have 3 sugar-free lemon sandwich cookies instead
Dinner			
Grilled chicken breast strips	3 ounces	4 ounces	5 ounces
Bulgur	1 cup	1½ cups	1½ cups, topped with ¼ cup walnuts
Steamed yellow squash	½ cup	½ cup	½ cup
Creamy French salad dressing, sugar free	1 tablespoon	2 tablespoons	2 tablespoons
Evening snack			
Low-fat frozen yogurt, sugar free (nonfruit flavor)	—	½ cup	1 cup
Walnuts	¼ cup	2 tablespoons	—

DAY 8

	1,200 CALORIES	1,600 CALORIES	2,000 CALORIES
Breakfast			
Cream of Wheat	1 cup	1½ cups	1½ cups
Low-fat milk (for Cream of Wheat)	—	¼ cup	½ cup
Sourdough bread, toasted	1 slice	1 slice	1 slice
Sesame tahini	1 tablespoon	1 tablespoon	1 tablespoon
Lunch			
Roasted turkey (for sandwich with next three items)	3 ounces	3 ounces	3 ounces
Rye bread	2 slices	2 slices	2 slices
Fresh avocado	¼ avocado	¼ avocado	⅓ avocado
Alfalfa sprouts	½ cup	½ cup	½ cup
Low-fat baked tortilla chips	10 chips	20 chips	25 chips
Afternoon snack			
Fudgsicle ice cream bar, sugar free	1	1	1
Dinner			
Baked potato stuffed with cheese and mushrooms (see below)	1 medium	1 medium	1 medium
Low-fat shredded Colby and jack cheese	¼ cup	⅓ cup	⅓ cup
Sliced mushrooms, sautéed in 1 tablespoon olive oil with 2 chopped garlic cloves	½ cup	½ cup	1 cup
Steamed kale	½ cup	½ cup	½ cup
Evening snack			
Almonds	—	¼ cup	¼ cup
Low-fat frozen yogurt, sugar free (not fruit flavor)	½ cup	—	1 cup

DAY 9

	1,200 CALORIES	1,600 CALORIES	2,000 CALORIES
Breakfast			
Low-fat breakfast sausage (pork or turkey)	2 links	2 links	2 links
Sourdough English muffin, toasted	1	1	1
Soft-spread margarine	1 teaspoon	1 teaspoon	2 teaspoons
Lunch			
Tricolored rotini (for pasta salad with other four ingredients)	1 cup	1½ cups	2 cups
Grilled chicken strips (precooked)	1 ounce	2 ounces	2 ounces
Fresh sliced mushrooms	½ cup	½ cup	½ cup
Sliced black olives	1 tablespoon	1 tablespoon	1 tablespoon
Light Italian dressing, sugar free	2 tablespoons	2 tablespoons	3 tablespoons
Afternoon snack			
Chocolate-vanilla swirl pudding cup, sugar free	1 snack cup	1 snack cup	Have 3 cups low-fat microwave popcorn instead
Fudge-striped shortbread cookies, sugar free	—	2	—
Dinner			
Broiled halibut	4 ounces	5 ounces	6 ounces
Basil pesto sauce, microwaveable	2 tablespoons	2 tablespoons	2 tablespoons
Couscous	½ cup	1 cup	1½ cups
Steamed green beans	½ cup	½ cup	½ cup
Evening snack			
Low-fat microwave popcorn	3 cups	—	—
Peanuts	—	¼ cup	¼ cup

DAY 10

	1,200 CALORIES	1,600 CALORIES	2,000 CALORIES
Breakfast			
Cheerios	1 cup	1 cup	1½ cups
Chopped walnuts	1 tablespoon	2 tablespoons	—
Low-fat milk	¾ cup	¾ cup	1 cup
Rye bread, toasted	—	—	1 slice
Soft-spread margarine	—	—	1 tablespoon
Lunch			
Boca Burger, original	1	1	—
Chicken breast, deli sliced	—	—	3 ounces
Tortilla	1 medium (about 7 inches in diameter)	1 medium (about 7 inches in diameter)	1 large (about 10 inches in diameter)
Lettuce leaf	1	1	1
Low-fat baked tortilla chips	13	20	25
Chunky salsa	2 tablespoons	2 tablespoons	2 tablespoons
Afternoon snack			
Chocolate-vanilla swirl pudding cup, sugar free	1 snack cup	1 snack cup	1 snack cup
Chopped walnuts	—	—	2 tablespoons
Dinner			
Beef (stir-fried with 1 or 2 chopped garlic cloves, ½ cup green cabbage, and ½ cup mushrooms)	3 ounces	4 ounces	4 ounces
White rice	¾ cup	1 cup	1½ cups
Evening snack			
Fudgsicle ice cream bar, sugar free	1	—	—
Low-fat frozen yogurt, sugar free (nonfruit flavor)	—	1 cup	1 cup

DAY 11

	1,200 CALORIES	1,600 CALORIES	2,000 CALORIES
Breakfast			
Sourdough baguette	1, about 6 inches long	1, about 6 inches long	1, about 6 inches long
Soft-spread margarine	1 teaspoon	1 teaspoon	—
Swiss cheese	—	—	1-ounce slice
Hot oatmeal	—	—	1 cup
Low-fat hot cocoa, sugar free	1 cup	1 cup	1 cup
Lunch			
Lentil soup	1 cup	1¼ cups	1½ cups
Rye bread	1 slice	1 slice	2 slices
Monterey Jack cheese	1-ounce slice	1-ounce slice	—
Soft-spread margarine	—	—	2 teaspoons
Fresh mixed salad greens	—	—	2 cups
Light Italian salad dressing, sugar free	—	—	2 tablespoons
Afternoon snack			
Fudge-striped short-bread cookies, sugar free	1 cookie	—	—
Almonds	—	¼ cup	¼ cup
Dinner			
Grilled chicken breast	3 ounces	4 ounces	5 ounces
Wild rice	1 cup	1 cup	1½ cups
Steamed cauliflower	½ cup	½ cup	½ cup
Light Alfredo sauce	¼ cup	¼ cup	¼ cup
Evening snack			
Low-fat microwave popcorn	3 cups	5 cups	—
Low-fat frozen yogurt, sugar free (nonfruit flavor)	—	—	1 cup

DAY 12

	1,200 CALORIES	1,600 CALORIES	2,000 CALORIES
Breakfast			
Shredded Wheat 'N Bran	1 cup	1½ cups	1½ cups
Toasted sunflower seed kernels	1 tablespoon	2 tablespoons	2 tablespoons
Low-fat milk	¾ cup	¾ cup	1 cup
Lunch			
Roast beef, deli sliced (for sandwich)	3 ounces	3 ounces	3 ounces
Sourdough bread	2 slices	2 slices	2 slices
Fresh celery	1 rib	—	—
Low-fat baked tortilla chips	—	20 chips	25 chips
Afternoon snack			
Lemon cream sandwich cookies, sugar free	2	3	3
Dinner			
Portobello mushroom, sautéed with 2 chopped garlic cloves in 1 tablespoon olive oil (for topping on fettuccine)	1 mushroom	1 mushroom	1 mushroom
Fettuccine	½ cup	1 cup	1½ cups
Low-fat shredded Cheddar cheese	¼ cup	¼ cup	⅓ cup
Fresh mixed salad greens	1 cup	1 cup	2 cups
Light Italian salad dressing, sugar free	2 tablespoons	2 tablespoons	2 tablespoons
Evening snack			
Chocolate-vanilla swirl pudding cup, sugar free	1 snack cup	1 snack cup	1 snack cup
Chopped walnuts	—	—	2 tablespoons

DAY 13

	1,200 CALORIES	1,600 CALORIES	2,000 CALORIES
Breakfast			
Scrambled egg	1 large	1 large	1 large
Home fries	½ cup	½ cup	1 cup
Rye bread, toasted	1 slice	1 slice	1 slice
Soft-spread margarine	1 teaspoon	1 teaspoon	1 teaspoon
Lunch			
Chopped chicken breast (for tortilla with next three items)	3 ounces	4 ounces	4 ounces
Corn tortilla	2, about 6 inches in diameter	4, about 6 inches in diameter	4, about 6 inches in diameter
Sliced black olives	2 tablespoons	2 tablespoons	4 tablespoons
Alfalfa sprouts	1 cup	1 cup	1 cup
Chunky salsa	2 tablespoons	2 tablespoons	4 tablespoons
Afternoon snack			
Fudge-striped shortbread cookies, sugar free	2	—	—
Low-fat frozen yogurt, sugar free (nonfruit flavor)	—	½ cup	1 cup
Chopped walnuts	—	1 teaspoon	1 tablespoon
Dinner			
White French bread pizza	1 serving	1 serving	1 serving
Fresh mixed salad greens	2 cups	2 cups	2 cups
Light Italian salad dressing, sugar free	2 tablespoons	2 tablespoons	2 tablespoons
Evening snack			
Fudgsicle ice cream bar, sugar free	1	—	—
Shredded Wheat 'N Bran	—	¾ cup	1½ cups
Low-fat milk	—	½ cup	¾ cup

DAY 14

	1,200 CALORIES	1,600 CALORIES	2,000 CALORIES
Breakfast			
Sourdough English muffin, toasted	1	1	1
Low-fat cream cheese	2 tablespoons	2 tablespoons	2 tablespoons
Low-fat hot cocoa, sugar free	—	1 cup	1 cup
Lunch			
Barley and mushroom soup	1 cup	1½ cups	2 cups
Reduced-fat Triscuits	7	10	12
Swiss cheese	½ ounce	1-ounce slice	1-ounce slice
Afternoon snack			
Lemon cream sandwich cookies, sugar free	2	—	—
Low-fat frozen yogurt, sugar free (nonfruit flavor)		1 cup	1 cup
Sunflower seeds	—	—	2 tablespoons
Dinner			
Grilled salmon	4 ounces	5 ounces	6 ounces
Baked potato	1 medium	1 medium	1 medium
Steamed green beans	½ cup	½ cup	½ cup
Light Italian salad dressing, sugar free	2 tablespoons	2 tablespoons	2 tablespoons
Evening snack			
Low-fat microwave popcorn	3 cups	—	—
Low-fat hot cocoa, sugar free	1 cup	—	—
Almonds	—	¼ cup	¼ cup

Phase II: The Low-Fructose Lifestyle

Calling the second stage of the Low-Fructose Diet a "phase" is a bit misleading, because it doesn't have a defined duration. Instead, I'm describing a way for you to eat for the rest of your life.

Now that you have successfully turned down the activity and reduced the volume of your fructose enzymes, you can resume a healthy—if limited—relationship with fructose. Your body will be able to handle modest amounts of sugar without slipping into the metabolic chaos that promotes weight gain and disease.

What exactly do I mean by "modest"? From now on, I want you to limit your fructose intake to 25 to 35 grams per day. If you eat a typical American diet, that's approximately one-third to one-half of the fructose you may be ac-

---

CASE STUDY: ELIMINATING HFCS, GAINING PROTECTION AGAINST DIABETES

Chuck Nelson (a pseudonym) had never been much of a soda drinker, but early in the summer of 2006, he began sipping carbonated soft drinks to quench his thirst while working in the garden. By July, Chuck noticed that he had put on several pounds. More worrisome, that same month he was diagnosed with type 2 diabetes, the condition that had claimed his father's life.

Chuck, 60, immediately switched to diet soda and decided to eliminate foods containing high-fructose corn syrup (HFCS) from his diet, which required some detective work. A ketchup lover, Chuck discovered from reading ingredient labels that most brands contain HFCS. (He did find a low-carb brand that's fructose free.) He was also surprised to find HFCS in some less likely foods, such as Italian salad dressing, bread—even "natural grain" varieties—and other foods that don't necessarily taste sweet. "Who'd have thought that horseradish sauce was made with HFCS?" asks Chuck.

His efforts have paid off. From a high of 216 pounds, Chuck has dropped down as low as 196 pounds. Better yet, he has lowered his risk for developing diabetes complications by maintaining his blood sugar in a healthy range.

customed to consuming every day. It's also the amount of fructose that I estimate most Americans consumed daily in the early 1900s—back when obesity, heart disease, and diabetes were rare conditions.

As you will see, 25 to 35 grams is a fairly generous fructose allowance that permits you to eat a balanced diet, including healthful fruits. It even allows you to splurge on an occasional sugary dessert, if you wish.

It is vitally important not to exceed 35 grams per day. If you do, you risk restarting the biological mechanisms that made you gain weight in the first place. To keep your daily fructose intake within a healthy range, you will need to become keenly aware of the total amount of fructose you eat.

To help you control your fructose intake, I have provided an appendix of tables that identify the fructose content of many common foods (see page 350). These tables categorize foods according to whether they have little or no fructose, or their content is low, moderate, or high. The tables are by no means comprehensive, but they can help you to estimate how much fructose you're getting from most of the foods that make up a typical diet. Here's how to use them.

- A wide range of foods contains natural and added sources of fructose, though in some cases, the amounts are very small. Start out by assuming that you will ingest 5 grams of fructose every day from miscellaneous foods.

- Consult the fructose tables when choosing foods from the following categories.
  Fruits
  Vegetables

Breads and Grains
Bread Toppings and Condiments
Salad Dressings
Breakfast Cereals
Beverages
Alcoholic Beverages
Sweeteners
Desserts and Dessert Toppings
Fast Foods

Your total fructose intake from these categories should be in the range of 20 to 30 grams.

- Your overall daily fructose intake should be between 25 and 35 grams.

- Pay close attention to the serving sizes listed in the fructose tables. If you eat a larger portion than what is specified, use your best judgment

CASE STUDY: CONTROLLING A CHILD'S TASTE FOR SUGAR

Elizabeth and Chris came to me out of concern for their 8-year-old son. At 4 feet 3 inches, he had already reached 100 pounds. I explained the basic concepts of the Low-Fructose Diet, and they decided to have the boy try it.

They replaced the sugary breakfast cereals their son had been eating with low-sugar varieties, sweetening them with Splenda. He was permitted only two or three pieces of fruit per week. Elizabeth and Chris stopped buying processed foods made with high-fructose corn syrup. They also eliminated fruit juice and fruit punches, as well as soft drinks, though their son was allowed to have diet soda.

Over the next 6 months, the boy lost 10 pounds, or 10 percent of his total body weight, despite growing 2 inches. He grew another 2 inches during the subsequent year, but gained only 6 pounds. Best of all, Elizabeth and Chris report that their son's appetite for sugary foods gradually declined.

to estimate how many grams of fructose to add
to your daily total.

Over time, as you become familiar with the fructose
content of your favorite foods, you will probably find that
you need to refer to the fructose tables only on occasion. It's
a sure sign that you are adapting to the Low-Fructose Lifestyle as you learn how to choose healthy foods and avoid
others that disrupt your metabolic balance.

The 12 Rules for Healthy Eating

I believe that the most important step you can take toward
a healthier, longer life is to limit your fructose intake. That
said, moderating the amount of sugar and HFCS you consume is merely the cornerstone of a sound nutrition plan.

As part of a Low-Fructose Lifestyle, I strongly recommend adopting the following simple rules for healthy eating. These commonsense guidelines are based on the
nutrition concepts I discussed in Chapter 9. Applying these
principles to your diet reduces your intake of foods and dietary elements that promote weight gain and disease—such
as purines, saturated and trans fats, and excess salt—while
increasing your intake of foods that can help you stay trim
and healthy.

1. Eat one or two servings of fruit daily. Once you
have completed the Fructose-Free Phase of my diet, eating
fruit is not only permitted but encouraged, provided you
limit yourself to one or two servings per day. Choose a variety of fruits, but be sure to include frequent servings of
those that are rich in vitamin C, such as oranges, grapefruit, and kiwifruit. Vitamin C reduces uric acid and may
help to lower blood pressure and control other conditions of

metabolic syndrome. In the table on page 350, you'll easily be able to identify fruits that are excellent sources of vitamin C by looking for the asterisk. (Cherries are a good choice, too; though moderately high in fructose, they seem to lower uric acid. See "A Reason to Cherish the Cherry" on page 165.)

On the other hand, beware of some old advice: An apple a day may not keep the doctor away after all, because the crisp fruit is rather high in fructose, as are pears and grapes. Eat these and other high-fructose fruits sparingly—no more than twice a week.

Another potential pitfall: most dried fruit, which has little or no vitamin C but is very high in fructose. A cup of dried figs, for example, contains nearly a day's worth of fructose. (One exception: A prune contains slightly more than 1 gram of the sugar.) Likewise, candied fruit isn't much better than candy. And canned fruit, such as mandarin oranges, is often steeped in sugary syrup.

Bear in mind that a small glass (4 to 6 ounces) of fruit juice counts as one serving of fruit; what many people consider a "serving" could be at least two, if not more. Also, certain varieties of juice, such as orange and apple, are extremely high in fructose. Unsweetened grapefruit juice and tomato juice are healthful, lower-fructose alternatives.

2. Pay attention to purines. Purines raise uric acid, so become familiar with foods that contain large amounts. The table on page 370 may be a helpful guide. In general, limit high-purine foods to once per month (with the exception of shrimp, which you can eat up to twice per month). As a rule, don't eat more than one serving of moderate-purine foods per day.

3. Eat four or five servings of vegetables per day.

Choose a variety of vegetables, making sure to include frequent servings of those that are low in fructose. (Use the table on page 350 as a reference.) Keep in mind that preparation methods can increase the fructose content. Avoid dishes such as glazed carrots and candied yams, as well as other recipes that call for sugar or honey. Avoiding fried vegetables is wise, too, because they are high in fat.

Some vegetables—such as asparagus, mushrooms, and cauliflower—are moderately high in purines. You don't need to avoid these varieties, but don't eat them every day, either. (Refer to the table on page 370 to learn which other vegetables are moderately high in purines.)

Aim for a total of four or five servings of vegetables every day. Remember that eating more vegetables than fruit will help you to avoid overloading your body with fructose.

4. Consume at least three servings of dairy foods and beverages per day. Dairy foods offer many health benefits. Studies have shown that consuming milk and other dairy products accelerates weight loss, perhaps in part because they lower uric acid. Choose low- or fat-free milk, low-fat cheese, low-fat plain (unflavored) yogurt, and other dairy foods. Whole-milk varieties are high in saturated fat, which increases the risk for heart disease.

Beware of processed dairy products that contain added sugar and HFCS, such as chocolate milk and fruit-flavored yogurt. Of course, ice cream is a dairy food, but it also contains a great deal of fructose, to say nothing of saturated fat.

5. Eat beef, pork, and lamb no more than two or three times a week. Favor lean cuts, such as sirloin or top round. Organ meats, such as liver, are high in purines. Eat them rarely, if at all. Be aware that condiments commonly served with meats, such as ketchup and barbecue sauce, can be stealth sources of fructose. Skinless chicken and turkey are excellent alternatives to red meat.

6. Eat fish at least twice a week. Fish is a rich source of omega-3 fatty acids, the healthy fats that can lower the risk for heart attack. But it also contains purines, which means that it has the potential to raise uric acid. Choose fish on the following basis.

- Cod, haddock, sole, and many other white-fleshed fish have lower purine content than most dark-fleshed fish. Eat them as often as you like.

- Salmon and tuna are moderately high in purines, but they also are among the top sources of omega-3 fatty acids. You can eat these fish once per week total.

- The following fish and shellfish are high in purines: anchovies, clams, herring, mackerel, mussels, sardines, oysters, scallops, lobster, and crab. Eat no more than one serving from this group per month. You can eat shrimp up to twice a month.

7. Eat six to eight servings of bread, cereal, rice, pasta, and other grains every day. Don't be tempted to skip starches because they are carbohydrates. The main sugar in bread and other starches, glucose, does *not* activate the mechanisms that cause insulin resistance and other conditions of metabolic syndrome. Furthermore, eating starchy foods will help prevent ketosis, the undesirable phenomenon that occurs in people who adopt diets that are very low in carbs.

During the Fructose-Free Phase, I ask you to avoid bread that contains 1 gram or more of fructose per serving. This includes whole wheat and whole grain products. Once you complete those first 2 weeks and your fructose enzymes are under control, it's not only safe but preferable to eat these varieties of bread, because they contain more fiber than bread made from refined grains.

8. Include healthy fats in your diet. Along with fatty fish, be sure to eat plenty of foods rich in beneficial mono-unsaturated fats, such as nuts, olive and canola oil, and avocados. Meanwhile, watch out for artery-clogging saturated fat, such as full-fat dairy products and fatty meats. (But— very important!—don't avoid dairy altogether; simply choose low-fat and fat-free foods, as explained earlier.)

Trans fat is even worse for you, and many commercial baked goods are full of the stuff (as well as fructose, in the case of cookies, cakes, and pies). French fries and other fast foods are other top sources of trans fat.

9. Don't eat excessive amounts of salt. If you do not have hypertension and you enjoy the taste of salt, feel free to sprinkle a little on food as you like—with the emphasis on "a little." The salt we add to food while cooking or at the dinner table accounts for about 15 percent of our sodium intake. A small amount occurs naturally in many foods; an 8-ounce glass of low-fat milk contains more than 120 milligrams, for example. But about three-quarters of the sodium in the American diet comes from processed foods. Canned soups and luncheon meats are among the saltiest products, which is a good reason to eat them sparingly.

10. Mind your condiments. Use condiments that contain added sugar or HFCS sparingly, if at all. Alternatives to sugar-laden sauces include:

- Yellow, brown, or horseradish mustard (avoid honey mustard)

- Wine or rice vinegar (read labels; some varieties contain sugar)

- Lemon juice

- Tabasco sauce

- Soy or tamari sauce (read labels; some varieties contain sugar)

Herbs and spices are fructose-free flavor enhancers. Combinations of spices known as "dry rubs," often used in Southern barbecue cooking, usually are fructose and calorie free—though they often contain a large amount of salt.

11. Reserve sugary desserts for special occasions. A large slice of chocolate cake can contain a day's worth of fructose. To keep your fructose enzymes under control, make sugary desserts a rare treat. When you do have a slice of cake or a bowl of ice cream, limit yourself to a small serving.

12. If you drink alcoholic beverages, avoid beer and those that contain sugar. Sorry, beer lovers, but your beverage of choice is a rich source of purines, which raise uric acid levels and may give you a beer belly, among other conditions of metabolic syndrome. Likewise, try to avoid cocktails made with nondiet soda, fruit juice, or other mixers that contain sugar or HFCS. Wine—ideally a dry variety—is the best option; avoid sweet wines, such as sherry, muscat, port, and Riesling. Though wine may have important health benefits, you should limit yourself to two glasses per day. (Remember, one glass of wine equals 5 ounces.)

The Next Steps

I wrote this book to show you how to achieve a healthy weight and lower your risk for devastating diseases by reducing your intake of sugar and HFCS, while making some other simple changes to your diet. But there is much you can do away from the dinner table to enhance the benefits of the Low-Fructose Diet.

In Part IV, I'll discuss other ways to fight the effects of fructose and bring your body back to metabolic balance. I'll also address questions and concerns that you may have before embarking on the Low-Fructose Lifestyle.

MAKE IT A BAKER'S DOZEN

One more rule of healthy eating: Enjoy your mealtimes. The Low-Fructose Diet may call upon you to make some changes in the way you eat, but that doesn't mean it should lose its pleasure. My colleague and collaborator, Elizabeth Gollub, PhD, has studied how dining habits affect a person's overall "nutritional quality of life." She offers the following suggestions.

- Think of mealtime as an opportunity to take a break and relax.

- Don't force yourself to eat foods you dislike; select only foods you enjoy.

- Make meals seem special by using attractive dishes and tableware. If you're having a glass of water with a meal, add a lemon wedge (which is very low in fructose, by the way). Presentation can make a difference.

- Eat with friends and family—unless you feel like eating alone.

- Turn off the television. You don't want to get in the habit of eating every time you pick up the remote control. Turn on some favorite music instead.

PART IV

MORE THAN A DIET: THE LOW-FRUCTOSE LIFESTYLE

CHAPTER 12

FURTHER STEPS

Complementing the Low-Fructose Diet

The Low-Fructose Diet is a powerful tool that will help you lose weight and correct metabolic problems that increase your risk for disease. As you'll soon see, you can take steps to make it work even better.

In this chapter, I'll outline a number of measures that will complement the diet you just read about. For example:

- We all know, of course, that regular exercise is a lifesaver. Getting off the sofa and working up a sweat specifically targets and minimizes one of the major forms of damage caused by eating too much fructose.

- Recognizing that you may already be dealing with elevated cholesterol, high blood pressure, and diabetes, I'll explain how common medications used to treat these conditions can

combat or—in some cases—*worsen* the
problems brought on by excess fructose.

- I also recognize that many people today seek
  out alternative cures for what ails them. I'll
  give you the facts about several natural
  treatments you may have read about that offer
  promise for reversing some of fructose's ill
  effects.

- Although I discussed diet and nutrition in
  Part III, I'll pass along a few more tips about
  foods that will enhance the effects of a
  low-fructose eating plan.

Many of the suggestions I am about to offer have benefits beyond their ability to counteract the fructose effect. While you may need to discuss some of these steps with your physician before you try them, nothing I am about to suggest is exotic, expensive, or hard to find. All will enhance the Low-Fructose Lifestyle.

Low-Fructose Lifestyle Recommendation: 30 Minutes of Moderate Physical Activity on Most Days

To the long list of reasons that you should exercise regularly, add another: Physical activity lowers uric acid. Studies show that the benefit of regular exercise can be quite significant, too, reducing blood levels of uric acid by 10 to 20 percent.

We aren't sure how regular exercise lowers uric acid, but it probably involves several different mechanisms. For example, physical activity increases blood flow to the kid-

DON'T OVERDO IT

Though regular exercise improves uric acid levels, they actually may rise *during* a workout. This may occur because of dehydration, because a person depletes his or her cells of stored energy, or because damaged and overexerted muscle is releasing DNA and RNA into the blood.

The rise in uric acid tends to be most severe in people who engage in strenuous, prolonged exercise, such as marathon running or cycling, or in any activity that results in severe overexertion. For example, scientists analyzed the blood of 38 men who competed in the Otztal Radmarathon, a day-long cycling race that requires a trek of 230 kilometers (about 138 miles) across the Austrian Alps. On average, the competitors' uric acid levels rose by 42 percent.

People who participate in marathon sporting events can largely protect themselves from these dramatic leaps in uric acid levels by drinking plenty of fluids. In fact, sports drinks that contain small amounts of fructose with electrolytes may be helpful in these circumstances (see Chapter 13).

neys, which in turn will increase the amount of uric acid you excrete in urine. Exercise also supports weight loss, which lowers uric acid levels, too.

Of course, there are many other reasons that you should set up and stick with a regular exercise plan. Burning off excess calories will complement the Low-Fructose Diet I described in the previous chapter. What's more, aerobic exercise—that is, any form of physical activity that increases your heart rate and gets you huffing and puffing a bit— protects the cardiovascular system, reduces blood pressure, and helps to combat insulin resistance.

Don't forget strength training, though. Weight lifting and other forms of resistance training not only help tone your body, they actually help fight disease. Studies show, for instance, that lifting weights makes muscle more sensitive to insulin, which will reduce the risk for diabetes.

About 60 percent of Americans get too little exercise,

according to the Centers for Disease Control and Prevention; one in four gets no exercise at all. If you have been on the sidelines or work out only sporadically, establishing an exercise routine will speed up weight loss and produce swift improvements in risk factors for metabolic syndrome, including a better uric acid profile.

It's always wise to talk to your doctor before embarking on a new fitness regimen, especially if you have an existing medical condition. In general, most experts agree that getting at least 30 minutes of moderately intense exercise (such as brisk walking) on all or at least most days is a good goal. Increasing the time you spend exercising will reap greater rewards (though longer, more intense workouts may raise the risk for injury).

For information about setting up your own exercise plan, check the Web site created by HealthierUS, an initiative of the US Office of Disease Prevention and Health Promotion (www.healthierus.gov).

Low-Fructose Lifestyle Recommendation: 10 to 15 Minutes of Sun Exposure, Twice a Week

As I explained in Chapter 10, new research suggests that vitamin D may combat certain serious health problems that arise when you eat a high-fructose diet. In particular, vitamin D suppresses the renin angiotensin system (RAS), a mechanism that raises blood pressure. The RAS can be activated when you eat too much fructose. This is one of several reasons that dairy products play such an important role in the Low-Fructose Diet: Most milk sold in the United States is fortified with vitamin D.

To be sure that you're getting adequate levels of this important vitamin, I strongly recommend spending some time in the sun. Your body manufactures vitamin D when the sun's ultraviolet rays strike exposed skin. That said, there is no need to become a bronzed sun worshipper. To produce adequate vitamin D, all you need is 10 to 15 minutes of sun exposure, twice a week. Be sure to leave your face, hands, arms, or back bare and sunscreen free for this brief period.

If you plan to remain outdoors for more than 10 to 15 minutes, apply sunscreen with a sun protection factor (SPF) of 15 or higher to your skin to safeguard against skin cancer. If you are unable to get out in the sun, be doubly sure to consume plenty of dairy products or talk with your doctor about vitamin D supplementation.

Low-Fructose Lifestyle Recommendation: 250 Milligrams of Vitamin C, Once a Day

Vitamin C is a vital complement to the Low-Fructose Diet for several reasons. The first is one that few people recognize: Vitamin C lowers blood levels of uric acid by increasing the amount of this compound that is passed in the urine. A 2005 study at Johns Hopkins University found that taking 500 milligrams of vitamin C every day for 2 months lowers uric acid by 0.5 mg/dl, on average—a valuable reduction.

Vitamin C is also a potent antioxidant, which means that it neutralizes free radicals and the damage they reap, known as oxidative stress. Many of the health problems brought on by eating too many foods that contain sugar and high-fructose corn syrup (HFCS)—weight gain, high blood pressure, kidney damage, and others—arise in part because large doses of fructose increase levels of free radicals in the body. Oxidative stress promotes heart disease, cancer, and other diseases and appears to play a role in obesity, too.

Boosting your body's antioxidant protection should help to offset some of fructose's unhealthy effects. Yet if you keep up with medical news, you may have your doubts. After all, haven't studies shown that antioxidants don't work?

Vitamin C is just one of a wide range of antioxidants. Many people take dietary supplements containing these various vitamins, minerals, and other related compounds despite lingering questions about their effectiveness. Indeed, the overall record for antioxidant supplements in formal research is somewhat dismal, with many studies failing to show that they provide any significant health benefits. In fact, an analysis that appeared in the *Journal of the American Medical Association (JAMA)* in 2007 determined that people who take certain antioxidant supplements—particularly vitamin A, vitamin E, and beta-carotene—actually have a higher death rate than people who don't take these antioxidants.

It's not clear why these antioxidant supplements fail—or worse—in formal research. It may be that fat-soluble antioxidants, such as vitamin E, are less effective than water-soluble antioxidants, such as vitamin C, in the watery environment inside cells. (Fat-soluble vitamins are those that dissolve in fat, while water-soluble dissolve in water.) Interestingly, the analysis in *JAMA* found no increased risk for death among people who take vitamin C supplements.

What's more, our research suggests that vitamin C targets health problems linked to eating too much fructose. For instance, studies have shown that laboratory animals

develop high blood pressure when fed a high-fructose diet—
yet their blood pressure remains normal if they receive vitamin C supplements, too. Other research suggests that
vitamin C may protect against the damaging effects of uric
acid on cells in fat tissue and in blood vessels.

Furthermore, population studies bolster the argument
that vitamin C plays a vital role in preventing metabolic
syndrome. Consider, for example, that people who have
high blood pressure and heart disease tend to have low
blood levels of vitamin C.

Because vitamin C appears to offset some of fructose's
damaging effects—among its other crucial roles in the
human body—be sure that you're getting enough of this important antioxidant every day. As I explained in the previous chapter, you must take a dietary supplement containing
250 milligrams of vitamin C during the Fructose-Free
Phase of the diet, because you won't be consuming any
fruit—the major source of this vital vitamin—during this
period. I recommend that you continue taking the supplement after you complete the Fructose-Free Phase. This is a
safe, inexpensive way to increase your body's antioxidant
protection and reduce your uric acid level. (Note: High
doses of vitamin C may increase the risk for kidney stones,
which is why I recommend taking only 250 milligrams a
day. However, I don't recommend taking vitamin C if you
have had kidney stones in the past.)

I don't recommend taking any other antioxidant supplements, such as vitamin E. Studies show that they probably
don't offer any protection against heart disease or other
health benefits, and I believe they do little to block the effects of a high-fructose diet.

Low-Fructose Lifestyle Recommendation: Frequent Servings of Potassium-Rich Foods

One of the best ways to counter fructose's damaging effects is to bolster your body's endothelial function. Endothelial cells line the inside of all blood vessels, including the inner walls of arteries and the interior of the heart. Healthy endothelial cells allow blood vessels to expand and contract as necessary to promote efficient blood circulation. When endothelial function is impaired—which can occur as fructose in the diet triggers cells to produce uric acid—blood pressure rises, cells become insulin resistant, and other bad things happen.

Consuming adequate amounts of potassium can help ensure that your endothelial cells remain healthy. Human studies have shown that potassium supplements lower blood pressure, while animal research shows that the supplements improve insulin resistance. But don't take potassium supplements unless your doctor tells you to, in which case, you will receive a prescription for potassium pills and be closely monitored. High blood levels of potassium can cause cardiac arrest, especially in people with kidney disease (and as many as 20 million Americans have some form of kidney problems, though many don't realize it).

Instead, fill your menu with foods that are rich in potassium. Fruit is one of the best sources, though you should limit yourself to two pieces per day in general (and none during the Fructose-Free Phase of the diet). Other good sources include:

- Asparagus
- Avocados

- Chocolate and cocoa

- Coffee

- Legumes, such as dried beans, peas, and lima beans

- Milk

- Mushrooms

- Nuts, especially peanuts, almonds, and pecans

- Potatoes and sweet potatoes

- Pumpkin

- Tomatoes

- Winter squash

Keep in mind that some of these foods also contain a fair amount of fructose, so once you move into the Low-Fructose Lifestyle phase of the diet, they will contribute to your daily allowance of 25 to 35 grams. Refer to the fructose tables beginning on page 350 for more information.

Low-Fructose Lifestyle Recommendation: Dark Chocolate, on Occasion

Though I'm not going to recommend stocking up on Hershey bars, some components of dark chocolate may actually neutralize fructose's effects. Evidence of this surprising benefit comes from an even more surprising source.

The San Blas Islands, off the coast of Panama, are home to the Kuna Indians. About 60 years ago, scientists discovered that members of this tribe have extraordinarily low blood pressure and rarely suffer heart attacks. Obesity is rare among the Kuna, too. Their secret? It could be the cocoa leaf.

The Kuna Indians' low blood pressure is all the more remarkable given that they eat very salty diets, which should raise their blood pressure. But Harvard researcher Norman K. Hollenberg, MD, PhD, found that the Kuna also drink large amounts—typically five or more cups per day—of a beverage made with cocoa leaves. As it happens, cocoa leaves are one of nature's richest sources of flavonoids, which are dark pigments in plant foods that act as antioxidants. Flavonoids also stimulate the release of nitric oxide, which relaxes blood vessels and promotes healthy blood pressure. In other words, it reverses endothelial dysfunction, which is one of the serious problems that arise when you eat fructose.

Cocoa, of course, is the critical ingredient in chocolate. Unfortunately, eating chocolate candy every day is not the secret to losing weight and conquering metabolic syndrome. For starters, chocolate usually contains a large amount of fructose-rich refined sugar or HFCS to balance cocoa's naturally bitter flavor. Furthermore, most chocolate on the market has been processed in a manner that strips away much of its flavonoid content.

Certain varieties—notably, bitter-tasting dark chocolate—may contain a reasonably high level of flavonoids. Very few brands have been adequately analyzed to determine their flavonoid content, so choosing chocolate that can lower your blood pressure and improve circulation is largely guesswork. Though I do not recommend eating any form of candy on a routine basis, a small piece of dark chocolate now and then may be a good choice if you crave an occasional sweet.

Low-Fructose Lifestyle Recommendation: Medication, If Appropriate

We know that elevated uric acid is one of the critical problems that arise when you eat a diet rich in fructose and purines. A number of drugs are available to treat other metabolic problems that have been linked to diet, such as elevated cholesterol and high blood pressure. So you may be wondering: Why don't we have a medication that lowers elevated uric acid?

The fact is, we do. We also have drugs that exert little or no influence on uric acid, but they do block the effects of fructose. (Other drugs actually *raise* uric acid, as you'll see.) For some people, medication may enhance the benefits of adopting the Low-Fructose Diet.

Let's start with the medications that are designed to lower uric acid. Doctors prescribe these drugs to treat gout. Some block the formation of uric acid, such as allopurinol (sold under the brand names Aloprim and Zyloprim) and a newer drug called febuxostat (which, as of this writing, is awaiting approval by the FDA). Other drugs increase the amount of uric acid excreted in urine. The most common of these is probenecid (Benemid).

Allopurinol is the medication of choice among doctors for lowering uric acid in gout patients. It is fairly effective, capable of lowering uric acid by 2 to 3 mg/dl—even more in some cases. So why not give this medication to people with elevated uric acid who don't have gout?

Though allopurinol is reasonably safe, it carries some

risks. Two to 3 percent of patients who take it experience side effects, usually a skin rash. Furthermore, about 1 of every 1,000 patients who take this drug develops a life-threatening condition known as allopurinol hypersensitivity syndrome, which causes severe skin pain and rash—even skin shedding—as well as liver failure and kidney failure. These risks must be balanced against the benefits of aggressively lowering elevated uric acid.

Keep in mind that adopting the Low-Fructose Diet will help to lower your uric acid. I recommend getting your levels checked before you start the diet, then again a month or two later. If your uric acid remains elevated—5.5 mg/dl or higher for men, 5.0 mg/dl or higher for women—your doctor should closely monitor you for conditions of metabolic syndrome, such as weight gain, high blood pressure, elevated triglycerides, and insulin resistance. If your uric acid is very high—8.0 mg/dl or greater—then I recommend talking with your doctor about the pros and cons of taking medication to lower uric acid.

This is not a simple decision, and there is no right or wrong answer. Clinical trials are under way—with more in the planning stages—to determine whether lowering uric acid with drugs can help people lose weight, lower blood pressure, reduce insulin resistance, and treat other conditions of metabolic syndrome. Some promising trials have already been completed, including our study showing that lowering uric acid improved blood pressure in adolescents with hypertension. It will be several years before we know the results of other ongoing studies, however.

I believe that some day, medication will become routine treatment for patients with elevated uric acid, in much the same way that we currently prescribe medication for patients with high cholesterol. But until we have more evidence from clinical trials, it's impossible to make blanket recommendations about using medications to lower uric acid.

What's right for you? Only you and your doctor can decide. Personally, if my uric acid was elevated, I would want to lower it. Based on what we have learned from animal studies, I believe that reducing uric acid protects against weight gain, cardiovascular disease, and other leading killers. First, I would cut back on fructose and purines. If that didn't do the job, I would be faced with a difficult decision. As a physician and scientist, I would not recommend taking drugs to lower uric acid unless a patient had gout. These medications are not approved for other uses, and we need more clinical trials to ensure that they benefit other conditions. Personally, though, I feel the weight of evidence against uric acid is so great that I would probably take medication if I had a uric acid level of 8.0 mg/dl or higher, especially if I had features of metabolic syndrome.

Gout drugs may be the most powerful pharmacological agents we have for lowering uric acid. As I have noted, other common medications can influence this important disease risk factor. If you have been eating a high-fructose diet or you are overweight, you may already be receiving drug treatment for other conditions of metabolic syndrome. If so, here are some special considerations.

If you have high cholesterol

A number of drugs lower cholesterol. The most effective by far is a group of prescription medications known collectively as statins, which have provided us with a powerful tool against heart disease. These important medications may be even more powerful than we originally realized. They not only lower cholesterol, but according to intriguing evidence, some statins may reduce uric acid levels, too.

Statin drugs are among the most widely prescribed medications in the world. Technically, they're called HMG CoA reductase inhibitors, but they are better known by their brand names, which include Lipitor (atorvastatin), Lescol (fluvastatin), Mevacor (lovastatin), Pravachol (pravastatin), Crestor (rosuvastatin), and Zocor (simvastatin). The American Heart Association advises doctors to consider prescribing a statin if a patient has LDL ("bad") cholesterol of 190 mg/dl or higher. However, the benchmarks are lower for patients who have high blood pressure or a family history of heart disease, who smoke cigarettes, or who have other risk factors for heart disease. For instance, if a hypertensive patient's father had heart disease and the patient's LDL cholesterol is 130 mg/dl or higher, he'll likely receive a prescription for a statin drug. For high-risk patients, the current goal of therapy is to reduce LDL cholesterol to 70 mg/dl or lower.

The statins lower LDL cholesterol levels by 20 to 60 percent, according to studies. They also combat conditions of metabolic syndrome by modestly reducing triglyceride levels and slightly increasing levels of HDL ("good") cholesterol.

There is a great deal of scientific interest in learning whether statins offer other medical benefits. Several studies suggest that one statin in particular, Lipitor, may be the best choice for people with elevated uric acid. A team of Greek investigators found that a group of patients with high cholesterol who started Lipitor therapy lowered their uric acid levels by more than 8 percent. Interestingly, the study's authors determined that every 1 mg/dl drop in uric acid from taking Lipitor resulted in a 24 percent reduction in the risk for heart attack. A second study comparing Lipitor with Zocor found that only the former lowered uric acid.

Although this research is preliminary, if you take another statin to control cholesterol, you may want to ask your doctor about switching to Lipitor.

If you have high blood pressure

Depending on the type of medication prescribed for high blood pressure, it may influence your ability to rein in the effects of fructose—for better or worse.

Thiazides

The class of hypertension drugs known as thiazide diuretics represented a major medical breakthrough when they were introduced in the 1960s. Hypertension often occurs because of a defect in the kidneys that interferes with their ability to remove sodium from the blood. Thiazides overcome this defect by increasing the amount of sodium that a patient passes in the urine.

Thanks to their ability to lower blood pressure, thiazides reduce the risk for stroke and heart failure. They are often the first drug prescribed to patients with hypertension. Currently, more than 5 million people in the United States take hydrochlorothiazide, the most common of the thiazides.

Although a number of other blood pressure drugs are on the market, many patients require thiazides for good blood pressure control. This is particularly true for patients who are African American, who are older, who have diabetes or kidney disease, or whose hypertension does not respond to other drugs.

Unfortunately, thiazides have a few troublesome side effects. In particular, these drugs lower blood levels of potassium while increasing uric acid. Given their effect on uric acid, thiazides—perhaps not surprisingly—are also known to raise triglycerides and blood glucose levels, induce insulin resistance, and increase the risk for diabetes. The possibility of these side effects is especially worrisome given that many people with hypertension who are treated with thiazides already have metabolic syndrome.

Furthermore, according to several studies, the rise in uric acid that occurs in people who take thiazides may offset some of the cardiac benefits that these drugs confer by lowering blood pressure. One study of elderly patients with hypertension who took thiazides found that half experienced a rise in uric acid of 1 mg/dl or more. While patients whose uric acid remained unchanged cut their risk for heart attack by 50 percent, the patients taking thiazides whose uric acid rose gained no protection.

To learn more about how the widespread use of thiazides may be affecting overweight Americans with high blood pressure who take the drugs, we studied the effects of thiazides in laboratory animals that had developed metabolic syndrome after we fed them a high-fructose diet. As we expected, the thiazides improved hypertension in the lab animals, though their blood pressure did not reach normal. Furthermore, their uric acid levels rose, their potassium levels fell, and all of the conditions of metabolic syndrome worsened.

When we gave allopurinol to the animals to lower their uric acid, their blood pressure fell into the normal range.

Their triglycerides and insulin resistance improved, too. Giving potassium—which, like allopurinol, can improve endothelial function (as explained earlier in this chapter)—to the animals also improved blood pressure and insulin resistance.

What does all of this mean? It suggests that thiazides may be a double-edged sword. While this commonly prescribed drug improves blood pressure by acting as a diuretic, it worsens metabolic syndrome by raising uric acid and lowering potassium. It's important to remember that we performed these studies on laboratory animals. A clinical trial funded by the National Institutes of Health will evaluate whether allopurinol can help lower blood pressure and block the side effects caused by thiazides in humans.

In the meantime, if you have hypertension and you take a thiazide diuretic, ask your doctor if it is the only medication that can control your blood pressure, because the existing data suggest that you may want to avoid these medications. Other diuretics, such as amiloride or aldactone, may be just as effective but won't produce such troubling side effects.

If a thiazide is your only option, keep a close eye on your uric acid level. If it is 8.0 mg/dl or higher, I recommend talking with your doctor about taking a medication to lower your uric acid, bearing in mind that you must weigh the risks and benefits I described earlier.

ACE inhibitors and ARBs

Two other classes of hypertension medications—ACE inhibitors and angiotensin receptor blockers (ARBs)—seem to complement the effects of a low-fructose diet. These drugs act on a peptide (a chain of amino acids) called an-

CAN HORMONES HELP?

Women tend to have lower uric acid levels until they reach menopause, when their levels rise to equal those of adult males. We believe that younger women have relatively low uric acid because the hormone estrogen stimulates the kidneys to pass large amounts of this compound in the urine. Having naturally low uric acid levels may help explain why premenopausal women suffer few heart attacks and rarely develop hypertension and kidney disease. Laboratory studies show that young female animals are better able to resist the effects of fructose than males and older females, probably because their high estrogen levels reduce uric acid.

Furthermore, when women who have reached menopause begin hormone therapy (HT), their uric acid levels often drop. So if you are a woman who has reached menopause, should you consider HT in order to control your uric acid? Probably not. No one has studied whether HT is an effective treatment for blocking the effects of fructose.

What's more, contrary to conventional wisdom about HT, a major study—the Women's Health Initiative—found that estrogen and estrogen-progesterone combinations don't guard against heart disease and may actually increase the risk for stroke in postmenopausal women. No one is sure why, though it could be that HT increases blood clotting or causes some other cardiovascular problem. There are many other ways to reduce your uric acid, so I don't recommend using HT for this purpose.

giotensin II, which recent research suggests plays an important role in cardiovascular disease, diabetes, and metabolic syndrome. (ACE inhibitors block the formation of angiotensin II, while ARBs block its activity.)

Studies have shown that giving these medications to laboratory animals that have been fed a high-fructose diet protects them from developing conditions of metabolic syndrome—not just high blood pressure but insulin resistance, too. What's more, other research shows that people with hypertension who take ACE inhibitors cut their risk for developing diabetes. Both drugs seem to protect the heart beyond their ability to lower blood pressure.

We're still trying to understand how these medications

provide such a broad range of benefits. Some of our studies have found that uric acid may raise blood pressure partly due to its effect on the renin angiotensin system; both ACE inhibitors and ARBs block many of the effects of elevated uric acid in laboratory animals. One ARB, losartan, actually lowers uric acid, though the effect is modest. If you are overweight and have hypertension or heart disease, I believe an ACE inhibitor or ARB should be the first line of therapy.

Prescription for the Future? Natural Supplements and the Low-Fructose Diet

You don't need a prescription to buy dietary supplements and other natural therapies. This doesn't necessarily mean that they are safe. Keep in mind, too, that any company can sell these nondrug therapies without rigorously testing them to confirm that they actually treat or cure a medical condition.

That said, some dietary supplements on the market today show promise for counteracting the effects of a high-fructose diet. Here are three that I think may one day prove useful as adjuncts to the Low-Fructose Diet, though we have much more to learn about how they work.

N-acetyl cysteine

N-acetyl cysteine (NAC) is an antioxidant that is sold as a dietary supplement. Studies have shown that NAC can improve insulin resistance, blood fats, blood pressure, and (to a lesser extent) body weight in laboratory animals that have been fed fructose.

Research indicates that like vitamin C, NAC blocks oxidative stress in fat cells and blood vessels that occurs as uric acid levels rise, though NAC appears to work in a different manner. These studies suggest that NAC may help neutralize the effects of fructose in humans. While NAC may prove to be a useful weapon against obesity and metabolic syndrome someday, I do not recommend taking these supplements until they have been adequately tested in clinical trials.

L-carnitine

L-carnitine is a compound found in cells throughout the body. It is sold as a dietary supplement, too. L-carnitine helps transport fatty acids into a cell's mitochondria, or power plant, so it plays an important role in creating energy.

Many foods provide L-carnitine, including dairy products, red meats, nuts, and seeds. In fructose-fed laboratory animals, L-carnitine supplements help them burn fat. L-carnitine also improves their insulin resistance and, to a lesser degree, lowers their body weight.

This research suggests that L-carnitine may offer similar protection to humans. Until we know more, however, I do not recommend taking L-carnitine supplements.

L-arginine

L-arginine is an amino acid essential in forming nitric oxide, which relaxes blood vessels, promoting healthy blood pressure and circulation. As you know, uric acid interferes with these processes by causing endothelial dysfunction. Our research shows that supplements of L-arginine can block some of the effects of uric acid in laboratory animals. Other promising clinical studies involving humans suggest that foods rich in L-arginine and L-arginine supplements may improve blood pressure and kidney function.

More research is needed before L-arginine supplements can be recommended. In the meantime, some healthy foods are excellent sources of this amino acid, including lentils and nuts (especially hazelnuts, walnuts, and peanuts). These foods contain a minimal amount of fructose and offer other valuable health benefits, so be sure to include them in your diet.

"Good" bacteria

Can bacteria help you lose weight? In recent years, a new concept has emerged in obesity research: Some evidence suggests that your weight is governed, to an extent, by the type of bacteria in your intestines. Specifically, certain bacteria may reduce calorie intake by eating some of the food you consume, preventing it from being absorbed.

Molecular biologist Jeffrey Gordon, MD, of Washing-

UP AND DOWN: OTHER INFLUENCES ON URIC ACID

Diet has a major influence on uric acid levels, but it is not the only factor. For example, pregnancy causes a drop in uric acid by increasing blood flow to the kidneys. Elevated uric acid may occur under other circumstances such as:

- Heatstroke

- Heart failure and other conditions that result in impaired oxygen delivery to muscles and other tissue

- Starvation-induced ketosis

- Cancer chemotherapy (the destruction of malignant cells releases DNA and RNA into the blood, eventually converting to uric acid)

- Genetics (your genes may cause your body to produce naturally high levels of uric acid or excrete less uric acid)

IN THE WORKS

My research group at the University of Florida is developing new ways to help doctors identify and treat patients who are vulnerable to the effects of fructose. Keep an eye out for the following.

A Fructose Tolerance Test

Doctors identify patients with diabetes by administering a glucose tolerance test. We are developing several tests that would analyze the activity of a patient's fructose enzymes. One test would measure how much a patient's blood levels of uric acid change after consuming a standard dose of fructose. Another would measure levels of these enzymes in a patient's white blood cells.

Fructokinase Inhibitors

We are working to develop a drug that would block the activity of fructokinase, or fructose enzymes. This would completely alter the way your body processes fructose. Some of it would pass in the urine, while the rest would be burned as energy in the same way your body metabolizes glucose—that is, safely, without generating harmful by-products.

ton University, introduced this novel concept. Dr. Gordon discovered that he could reduce a mouse's body weight by converting its intestinal bacteria from one variety (known as Firmicute) to another (called Bacteroidetes). Dr. Gordon later showed that obese people have predominantly Firmicute bacteria in their intestines.

It's conceivable that fructose influences the type of bacteria in your gut, though we can't be sure of that. There is intriguing evidence that healthy bacteria may partially reverse some of fructose's ill effects. In one study, Indian researchers gave a type of fermented milk known as dahi to fructose-fed diabetic laboratory rats. Dahi contains strains of bacteria called *Lactobacillus acidophilus* and *Lactobacillus casei*. Compared with a group of rats that didn't receive the healthy bacteria, the rats fed dahi showed improved insulin resistance and blood fats.

Chances are, your local grocer does not stock dahi in the dairy case. On the other hand, yogurt is a readily available fermented milk product. I strongly encourage you to consume three servings of dairy foods every day. If you enjoy yogurt, you may want to seek varieties that contain these healthy bacteria, which will be identified on the label (though you still should avoid or limit fructose-sweetened varieties). I can't say that the healthy bacteria will help, but because dairy lowers uric acid, these foods certainly won't hurt.

CHAPTER 13

GOOD QUESTIONS

. . . And Some Final Thoughts About the Low-Fructose Diet

Over the past few years, I have spent a great deal of time giving lectures about the Low-Fructose Diet to groups of physicians and scientists around the United States and in other countries. My talks have been well received and are always followed by a spirited question-and-answer session. I've had the pleasure of discussing my research on fructose before lay audiences, too, and I never cease to be amazed by their insightful inquiries about the diet.

I'll bet by now you have a few questions of your own. In this chapter, I'll try to anticipate your lingering doubts or concerns about the Low-Fructose Diet by responding to some of the questions I have heard since I began studying its benefits.

Is fructose all bad?

No. In fact, fructose is an important part of the human diet. But think of it in the same way you would a drug:

Small amounts of fructose offer clear benefit, while consuming too much may make you sick. As the old saying goes, the dose makes the poison.

Fructose's most obvious upside is that it adds sweetness to fruit. This makes fruit more palatable, which increases our desire to eat these healthful foods. Try to imagine what an orange would taste like without fructose. With no sweetness to balance the sourness of citric acid, it would be too tart to eat, robbing our diets of a plentiful source of vitamin C, folic acid, and other essential nutrients. To a lesser extent, fructose adds flavor to vegetables, too.

Many scientific studies suggest that diets rich in fruits and vegetables fight disease and promote a longer life. Plant foods not only are rich in fiber, vitamins, and minerals, they also are chock-full of so-called phytochemicals, which function as antioxidants, fight inflammation, and promote health in myriad other ways. Thanks to fructose, fruits and vegetables are more appealing and therefore easier to swallow.

Fructose may offer additional benefits to athletes and other people who engage in intense physical exertion. During a long bout of exercise, the body burns a large amount of carbohydrate stored in the muscles and liver as fuel. Fatigue sets in, and performance falters as these reserves dry up. Studies have shown that giving beverages or other supplements that contain glucose to athletes during a long workout increases stamina and improves performance. But the amount of carbohydrate that can be burned as energy seems to peak at about 1 gram per minute.

This is where fructose may help. Several studies have shown that adding fructose to sports drinks increases the speed at which the body can absorb and burn glucose as fuel. For example, in one 2004 study by researchers at the University of Birmingham in the United Kingdom, eight trained cyclists were given different sports drinks as they pedaled stationary cycles for several hours. While drinking a solution that contained fructose and glucose, the cyclists increased the amount of carbohydrate they burned to 1.3 grams per minute and produced 55 percent more energy than when they drank a glucose-only beverage.

Obviously, the ability to produce more energy increases durability and improves athletic performance. Combining fructose and glucose also increases fluid absorption, which helps to prevent dehydration. In other words, a mix of fructose and glucose may allow athletes to compete harder, longer.

Many people seem to understand this fructose advantage intuitively. For example, nomadic Bedouins in desert regions have historically relied on dried figs and dates—both rich sources of fructose—during long treks across the sand. Likewise, many hikers today stock their backpacks with trail mix (also known as gorp), a high-energy blend of nuts, seeds, and fructose-rich dried fruit.

Interestingly, other studies have shown that supplementing the body with pure fructose actually results in worse performance. This makes sense, because—as I explained earlier—fructose causes cells to burn up their energy rapidly.

A sports drink should contain no more than 5 to 8 grams of fructose per serving. And these energy-replacement beverages are definitely not a good choice for nonathletes. For the couch potato watching a ball game on television at home, gulping down a sports drink is just another way to increase your overall fructose intake and offers no other health benefit.

What about people with diabetes? Isn't fructose a safer choice than table sugar?

Granulated fructose, which is available in health food stores and online, has earned a reputation in some circles as a healthier alternative to table sugar thanks to one of its unique qualities. When you consume fructose, your blood sugar levels don't rise suddenly. By contrast, the glucose in table sugar is absorbed rapidly into the bloodstream, causing levels of blood sugar to soar. Chronically elevated blood sugar can damage organs, so the body responds by taking action to lower blood levels of glucose. Beta cells in the pancreas produce the hormone insulin, which enters the bloodstream and triggers changes in cell membranes that allow glucose to enter cells. There glucose can be stored or burned as energy.

By contrast, your body doesn't need insulin to store fructose; most of it goes straight to the liver. This important distinction between fructose and glucose is of particular interest to people with diabetes. In type 1 diabetes, the pancreas produces no insulin, while people with type 2 diabetes aren't able to burn glucose efficiently because the cells in their body have become resistant to insulin. Because they lack an adequate insulin response, people with diabetes often avoid sweet foods, because their bodies are ill-equipped to process glucose. Several studies have shown that substituting fructose for table sugar in the diet helps people with diabetes maintain safe blood glucose levels. In fact, research suggests that adding a small amount of fructose to the diet may improve glycemic control by causing the liver to take up glucose faster, which means less enters the bloodstream.

Still, doctors no longer advise patients with diabetes to sweeten foods with fructose. The American Diabetes Association began discouraging the practice following the discovery that a high-fructose diet causes a rise in blood fats called triglycerides, which can clog arteries. As we now know, fructose can cause hypertension, vascular disease, and inflammation. Our research further shows that consuming too much fructose causes and worsens kidney disease. It also increases levels of compounds called advanced glycation end products, which may cause diabetic complications, including eye and kidney disease. These threats outweigh any benefit that a diabetes patient may get from using fructose as a sweetener.

What if I don't lose weight on the Low-Fructose Diet?

The vast majority of people who adopt the Low-Fructose Diet will lose weight rapidly. If your weight does not change much, one explanation may be that eating a very low-fructose diet for the initial 2-week phase failed to turn down the activity of your fructose enzymes. This may be because you inherited unusually high levels of these enzymes, or your enzymes are highly active. Or it could be that something in your environment other than fructose— something we have not yet identified—may be increasing your fructose enzymes.

Of course, if you didn't stick with the diet and you slipped in a few candy bars or bottles of soda, you may have compromised your weight-loss efforts. Our research shows that fructose enzymes are supersensitive and require a true fructose fast to turn down their activity.

My first piece of advice would be to repeat the 2-week Fructose-Free Phase a second time. If you did not choose the low-calorie option originally, you may want to give it a try now. In fact, you may want to consider repeating the 2-week Fructose-Free Phase every 6 months or so to help keep your fructose enzymes in check and maintain your weight at a desirable level.

Next, take a close look at your overall diet. Consuming too much fructose is a major cause of obesity—but it's not the only cause. Calories matter, of course, so if you are simply eating too much food and not exercising enough (or at all), you may continue to be overweight even if you swear off fructose. If this is the case, then you should strongly consider trying the low-calorie version of the Fructose-Free Phase and starting a regular exercise program if you haven't adopted one already. Once you have lost weight, sticking with the Low-Fructose Diet will help you keep off the weight, because a low fructose intake will help prevent insulin resistance and other hormonal changes that trick your body into regaining those unwanted pounds.

If cutting back on fructose does not help you lose weight, you may want to ask your doctor to check you for diabetes. Your doctor may recommend an oral glucose tolerance test, which screens for diabetes.

Because the Low-Fructose Diet is high in carbohydrates, it may not be ideal for people who are diabetic. But it can still be helpful, with some modifications. If you have diabetes, you should combine the concepts I've described in this book with the basic principles of the glycemic index (GI), which I discussed in Chapter 8. The GI was specifically designed for people with diabetes. Favoring low-GI foods will help you to maintain healthy blood glucose.

You cite a number of animal studies in this book. Are the findings from these studies relevant to humans? After all, in most cases, the animals consumed extremely large amounts of fructose.

Many studies have shown that feeding large amounts of fructose to laboratory animals causes them to become obese and develop other conditions of metabolic syndrome. In these studies, animals have often been fed diets in which up to 60 percent of the calories come from fructose. Skeptics have argued that these studies don't tell us anything about the effects of fructose on humans, because most people consume far less of the sugar. The typical American gets about 12 percent of his or her calories from fructose, although some people consume much more.

It's common to use large doses in experimental research in order to produce prompt results. It's possible, for example, to induce metabolic syndrome in a laboratory rat in less than 2 months. Furthermore, research has shown that feeding lab animals smaller amounts of fructose—35 percent of total calories—produces a milder form of metabolic syndrome. Giving lab rats a load of fructose proportional to what many Americans consume causes a key aspect of metabolic syndrome—insulin resistance—in a little over a year.

Another point: Animals may require larger doses of fructose because they have relatively low levels of uric acid, which drives many of fructose's ill effects. Our research shows that as we artificially increase uric acid in laboratory animals, they become more sensitive to lower doses of fructose.

Finally, bear in mind that animal research is only the beginning. We have ample experimental data to show that giving humans large daily doses of fructose or sucrose (which is half fructose) quickly causes weight gain, raises blood pressure and triglycerides, and induces insulin resistance.

I can understand why it's important to avoid soda, candy, and other high-fructose foods during the Fructose-Free Phase of your diet. But do I really need to avoid foods that contain even small amounts of fructose, too?

We can't say for sure—but why take the chance?

It is certainly possible that the cells in your body may be able to process small amounts of fructose without withstanding the kind of damage that makes them fat, become inflamed, and develop oxidative stress. The key question is this: Are your fructose enzymes elevated and overactive? If not, you could be okay. But if you do have high levels of very active fructose enzymes, then consuming even modest amounts of fructose might injure your cells and generate uric acid, which will set in motion the processes that lead to weight gain and other metabolic problems.

Unfortunately, we have no way of measuring whether your fructose enzymes are currently raging out of control—not yet, anyway. My colleagues and I hope to develop a fructose tolerance test, which would measure how fructose enzymes respond to a standard amount of the simple sugar. We are also working on a blood test that will measure the levels of fructose enzymes in your white blood cells.

For now, the safest and most effective way to ensure

that your fructose enzymes are not causing health problems is to bring them back to a healthy baseline by eliminating as much fructose as possible for the first 2 weeks of the Low-Fructose Diet. Once you have completed this fructose fast, your body will be able to manage modest amounts (25 to 35 grams per day).

My uric acid is low. Does that mean I have nothing to worry about?

Not necessarily. We know that eating fructose causes uric acid to rise. This makes the amount of uric acid in your blood a useful marker of how much damage fructose may be doing in your body. Still, the uric acid in your blood may be just the tip of the iceberg, so to speak, in that it represents only what has spilled out of your cells. The unmeasurable uric acid that remains inside your cells, along with other by-products of fructose metabolism, may still do damage. For this reason, even if your uric acid is not terribly high, you may be harming yourself by eating a high-fructose diet.

I have elevated uric acid, but I am slender and have normal blood pressure. If uric acid is so evil, then why am I so healthy?

It is undeniably true: Not everyone who has high uric acid will become fat or develop metabolic syndrome. Why? There are several possible explanations.

For instance, we know that uric acid seems to cause problems by reducing the amount of nitric oxide released by endothelial cells in blood vessels. As a result, blood vessels can't expand adequately—the problem known as endothelial dysfunction—which raises blood pressure and impairs circulation. But you may be resistant to the effects of uric acid because you exercise regularly, take vitamin C, or eat an antioxidant-rich diet. All of these measures strengthen endothelial function. Furthermore, some people simply inherit good endothelial function in their genes, which could negate the damaging effects of high uric acid.

Still, I encourage you to adopt the Low-Fructose Diet even if you feel fine and your weight is normal, especially if your uric acid is already elevated. Our studies suggest that over time, high uric acid can trigger changes in the body that lead to weight gain and other metabolic problems. Epidemiological studies confirm that people who have elevated uric acid are at increased risk for becoming seriously overweight and developing hypertension and insulin resistance—even if they are thin now. What's more, we know that a high-fructose diet harms the body beyond its ability to raise uric acid.

Some critics claim that high-fructose corn syrup, or HFCS, is largely responsible for the obesity epidemic. Should HFCS be banned?

Most people who consume too many foods sweetened with HFCS are going to have health problems. They will likely struggle with their weight and run the risk of developing other conditions of metabolic syndrome. But the same is true if you consume too many foods sweetened with refined sugar. Consider, after all, that obesity rates are rising worldwide—including in nations where foods made with HFCS are not available. On the other hand, studies consistently indicate that people are getting fatter in countries where the *total intake of sweeteners*—including HFCS and refined sugar—is rising.

So if we were to ban HFCS, it would only make sense to also ban refined sugar, the other major source of fructose in the American diet. At the same time, we would probably need to ban honey, which has more fructose by weight than either HFCS or refined sugar. Of course, none of this is likely to occur. The alternative is to carefully manage your consumption of foods that contain these sweeteners. The Low-Fructose Diet will help you do just that.

Much of the controversy over HFCS stems from the widespread perception that it is more dangerous than refined sugar. While this matter deserves scientific scrutiny, we simply do not know yet if it's true. The fructose and glucose in HFCS are not bound together the way they occur in refined sugar, or sucrose. In theory, this means that consuming foods or beverages sweetened with HFCS may produce higher blood levels of fructose. In turn, HFCS may be more likely to activate all of the unhealthy effects that we associate with a high-fructose diet, such as obesity and high blood pressure.

On the other hand, it's possible that blood levels of fructose simply rise faster immediately after you consume a product sweetened with HFCS, but the overall effect of consuming HFCS is the same as for sugar. Or, because sugar must be broken up by enzymes before it is absorbed, in theory, it could produce longer, sustained elevations in fructose, with worse effects.

Because none of these theories has been adequately tested, at this point, we can't say whether HFCS is any better or worse than refined sugar.

I have heard that some traditional folk healers recommend honey—which is extremely high in fructose—as medicine. How could this be?

Indeed, honey has been prescribed to treat a variety of conditions, including infections. It has also been recommended as a general immune system stimulant. This isn't surprising, because honey has a very high concentration of fructose, which triggers the release of inflammatory chemicals and oxidants. In theory, this might enhance the body's ability to fight infection.

To date, honey's medicinal value has not been well studied. But let's assume that honey does, in fact, stimulate inflammation. While this might be a good thing in the case of an acute infection, chronically stimulating the pathways that produce inflammation may not be. After all, we have powerful evidence showing that obesity, hypertension, and cardiovascular disease are all, to some extent, conditions that arise from chronic inflammation.

If you like honey, feel free to add some to your tea or include it in a recipe, though at nearly 9 grams of fructose per tablespoon, it takes a big bite out of your daily fructose budget. At this time, I can't recommend using honey for medicinal purposes.

If uric acid is so bad for us, why did humans lose the ability to make uricase, the enzyme that protects most other animals from its damaging effects?

Around 15 million years ago, our primate ancestors lost the ability to produce the enzyme uricase, which degrades uric acid, rendering it harmless. While I believe that high uric acid poses a serious health risk for modern humans, some scientists theorize that losing uricase allowed us to become Earth's dominant species. Let me explain.

Among uric acid's many intriguing and troublesome qualities, here is one I have mentioned just briefly: It is chemically similar to caffeine, the bitter-tasting compound in coffee, tea, and other foods and beverages that stimulates the central nervous system and promotes alertness. Some scientists believe that uric acid stimulates the central nervous system, too, and may have played a critical role in our development. It's conceivable, they argue, that by arousing the brain, excess uric acid contributed to the emergence of intelligence in humans.

This theory is supported by some intriguing observations. For instance, we know that high levels of uric acid cause gout. Although gout afflicts about 2 percent of the population, the condition has seemed—at least anecdotally—to occur with unusual frequency in people (usually men) of high achievement. Consider this short list of known gout sufferers throughout history: Alexander the Great, Charlemagne, Henry VIII, Benjamin Franklin, Alexander Hamilton, Alfred Tennyson, Samuel Coleridge, Voltaire, Leonardo da Vinci, Isaac Newton, and Charles Darwin.

Furthermore, some research has linked uric acid levels to intelligence and academic performance. For example, studies of high school students and military recruits found that people with elevated uric acid levels tend to score well on standard IQ tests. In one study, medical students who excelled in oral exams had relatively high uric acid.

In fairness, the relationship between uric acid and intelligence in these studies has been statistically significant, though not particularly strong. More persuasive is research linking high uric acid to admirable character traits, such as goal-oriented behavior, motivation, and leadership. Some studies suggest that elevated uric acid levels improve reaction time, too. Nevertheless, while acute rises in uric acid may offer some short-term benefits, we know that chronically high uric acid is associated with mental decline, as I explained in Chapter 7.

Others have argued that elevated uric acid may have protected the health of early humans, because it can act as an antioxidant. These defender compounds scavenge free radicals, which are molecules that promote disease and aging by damaging proteins and DNA. While uric acid is a relatively weak antioxidant overall, it is particularly effective at deactivating peroxynitrite, a free radical that is thought to play a significant role in damaging body tissue.

One theory goes like this: Early mammals were able to synthesize another important antioxidant, vitamin C. But our primate ancestors lived in tropical rain forests, where they had plenty of fruit to eat—and therefore were getting large amounts of vitamin C from their diets. Because their bodies didn't need to produce vitamin C, they eventually quit making it—that is, they developed a genetic mutation that eliminated the enzyme responsible for producing vitamin C. There is evidence that this mutation occurred 35 to 55 million years ago.

By the mid-Miocene era, however, climate changes caused many of the rain forests to disappear, which meant that far less fruit was available. To compensate for the loss of vitamin C, primates underwent another genetic mutation, losing the uricase enzyme. And so their uric acid levels rose, restoring antioxidant protection, too.

I have another hypothesis. When the rain forests began drying out, our primate ancestors were forced to travel across savannahs searching for food. This placed them at risk for dehydration and excessively low blood pressure, which was particularly true because what little food was available appears to have been very low in salt. For these reasons, a genetic mutation that led to higher uric acid levels could have been an advantage, because it would have helped our primate forebears by retaining salt and raising their blood pressure. High uric acid may have increased their body weight, too, allowing them to survive when food was scarce.

Unfortunately, modern humans—with our relatively high uric acid and our inability to synthesize vitamin C—are left vulnerable. Today's typical diet is full of fructose- and purine-rich foods, which raise uric acid to levels that are likely higher than those of primitive humans. While mildly elevated uric acid may have conferred benefits to early humans who struggled to get enough food to survive, the higher levels that are common today—brought on by diets full of high-fructose and high-purine foods—may be driving the current epidemic of obesity, high blood pressure, and heart disease. Combined with other poor dietary habits and lack of exercise, high uric acid—which once may have been a boon to human health—is now a major problem.

If uric acid is an antioxidant, doesn't that mean it should be good for me?

For a long time, many scientists believed that uric acid was biologically inert—a harmless, inactive by-product of energy metabolism that passed uneventfully out of the body. Then about 25 years ago, scientists discovered that uric acid is actually one of the body's important antioxidants. To explain why people with cardiovascular disease had high uric acid, some scientists suggested that it was simply the body's attempt to control the oxidative stress damaging the heart.

My group and other investigators have found the uric acid story to be much more complex. In some cases, uric acid is indeed beneficial, capable of neutralizing certain free radicals that would otherwise damage cells. But as I have explained, uric acid also depletes nitric oxide, which causes blood vessels to constrict, leading to high blood pressure and other problems. Uric acid generates free radicals, too. These effects, I believe, explain why high uric acid causes cardiovascular disease.

Still, scientists from a variety of disciplines are exploring whether uric acid has therapeutic value given its power as an antioxidant. Interest is particularly intense among my colleagues in the field of neurology.

For instance, several studies have shown that uric acid may play some role in treating or preventing multiple sclerosis. In fact, it's possible that one reason young women are unusually vulnerable to this devastating disease is that they have naturally low uric acid levels. Animal studies suggest that infusions of uric acid may help treat multiple sclerosis. Ironically, the very action that makes high uric acid so dangerous throughout the body—interfering with endothelial function, which prevents blood vessels from dilating—could have a silver lining. It's possible that high uric acid constricts tiny blood vessels in the brain, keeping white blood cells from entering and causing the tissue damage that leads to multiple sclerosis. Low uric acid has also been linked to an increased risk for Parkinson's disease.

There remains much to learn about the link between uric acid and these neurological diseases. For now, the well-established downsides of elevated uric acid outweigh its potential benefits as a preventive.

Have all studies shown that consuming large amounts of fructose causes obesity, hypertension, and other conditions of metabolic syndrome?

While the research linking fructose to obesity and other health problems is impressive, it's true that some studies have failed to indict this simple sugar. In particular, not all studies have shown that consuming fructose raises triglycerides or causes insulin resistance. There are many possible explanations for this.

For example, studies sometimes fail to show that fructose has much effect on healthy premenopausal women. In fact, we know that younger women are less susceptible to the effects of fructose than males are. But over time, if a woman eats a high-fructose diet, her fructose enzymes are very likely to rise and become overactive. Eventually, her body's natural resistance to fructose will be overwhelmed, and she will become more sensitive to its effects. Furthermore, we know that a steady diet of fructose-rich foods and beverages raises uric acid. Interestingly, some studies suggest that women are more sensitive to uric acid than men are and that when a woman's uric acid rises, it's more likely to cause high blood pressure, heart disease, and kidney disease. This all suggests that even a healthy young woman is likely to develop these complications if she consumes too much fructose.

The same thing may apply to the people who volunteer for scientific studies, who are often slender and healthy. Chances are, these individuals have good endothelial function and low levels of fructose enzymes. That will allow them to resist fructose's effects, at least initially. Giving healthy people small amounts of fructose, for the brief duration of a typical scientific study, is unlikely to show any effect.

Nor would such a study reflect what's happening in our society, where many people eat large amounts of fructose every day. It doesn't happen overnight, but if a person eats a typical Western-style diet, sooner or later his fructose enzymes rise, his uric acid creeps upward, and he becomes increasingly sensitive to fructose and all of its unhealthy effects. Indeed, clinical studies show that obese people are the most sensitive to fructose's effects because they usually have high levels of overactive fructose enzymes.

The overall weight of the evidence is clear: The more fructose you consume, the more your enzymes will rise and the more sensitive you will become. If you continue to eat a high-fructose diet, you will increase your risk for becoming overweight and developing high blood pressure, insulin resistance, diabetes, and other health problems.

How do you know that the Low-Fructose Diet works?

I've seen firsthand that everyone who tries this diet loses weight and keeps it off. My group plans to compare the Low-Fructose Diet to the Atkins plan and the DASH diet in a formal study. But I already know that we have developed a safe, effective approach to weight management and better health.

In recent years, studies have shown that low-carbohydrate diets can be an effective weight-loss option. The Low-Fructose Diet offers all of the benefits of a low-carb plan by targeting the *right* carbohydrate—fructose—which research has identified as a major cause of obesity and metabolic syndrome. The Low-Fructose Diet is more palatable than most low-carb plans, given the broader range of foods it allows. It's more nutritionally balanced, too, because it does not overemphasize protein or fat.

Many veterans of low-carb diets will wonder: How can I lose weight while eating so much starch? No need to worry. Studies clearly demonstrate that bread, potatoes, and other starchy carbohydrates are not obstacles to weight loss.

In one comparison study, overweight people were placed on a high-sugar, high-starch, or high-fat diet for 2 weeks. The people who followed the high-sugar and high-fat diets consumed the most calories and gained weight; those on the high-starch diet lost weight. This study suggests that starchy foods are less likely than sugary foods to make you fat.

I believe the reason that low-carb diets work is that they reduce fructose intake. By allowing you to eat bread, potatoes, and other well-loved foods, the Low-Fructose Diet encourages a normal balance of carbohydrates, making it a plan that most people can easily stick with for life.

CHAPTER 14

EPILOGUE

The last page of a novel often leaves the reader with a sense that even though the narrative has ended, the story is really just beginning. I feel the same way about this book. I have done my best in these pages to explain what we currently know about fructose, uric acid, and your health. But the story is far from over, and we still have much to learn.

Over the past century, obesity, cardiovascular disease, and many once-rare conditions have become the leading causes of death and disability in the United States and many parts of the world. In recent years, we have discovered new ways to treat people who develop these modern medical conditions. But patients often require medication, surgery, and other serious interventions that carry their own risk of side effects and burden our health-care system. Without a doubt, we must learn how to prevent these ailments from developing in the first place.

We have made progress in this regard. Although it seems obvious today, the earliest recognition that eating a typical American diet could make people fat and sick was a major breakthrough. The theory that dietary fat itself is the culprit appeared compelling initially, but the scientific data never fully supported that hypothesis. Proponents of low-carbohydrate diets offered a new way to bring down rampant obesity and disease rates. Studies suggest that these diets can produce significant weight loss and improve some conditions of metabolic syndrome. But low-carb diets are difficult to sustain and may not be safe, because they require people to eat unnaturally high amounts of protein and fat.

We now know that reducing intake of one particular carbohydrate, fructose, may be the key. The Low-Fructose Diet overcomes many of the problems found with other dietary approaches to weight loss and better health. It is backed by solid science, it's easy to follow, and it provides a healthy balance of carbohydrates, protein, and fat.

Many mysteries remain about how sugar, high-fructose corn syrup, and other sources of fructose affect health. Much of the evidence we have today comes from studies of laboratory animals. While more and more clinical trials are emerging to support the theories that I have presented in this book, it is of utmost importance that we confirm these findings with additional studies in humans. My group at the University of Florida is continuing on this path. It is my hope that the ideas and science I have discussed in these pages inspire other investigators to join us.

Despite the need for more study, the overall case against fructose and uric acid is overwhelming. The growing body of scientific evidence makes a powerful argument that a high-fructose diet is a major influence on the current epidemics of obesity, cardiovascular disease, and other conditions linked to metabolic syndrome. I feel that the Low-Fructose Diet offers the new approach we need to battle these health threats.

It is my belief that millions of lives could be saved if more people reduced their exposure to fructose. But you are probably wondering: What can I expect for myself? What will adopting the Low-Fructose Diet do for me? What's the payoff if I start looking for fructose in the ingredient lists of food labels? How is cutting back on sugary foods and beverages going to improve my health?

I have no doubt that just about anyone who is consuming a high daily dose of fructose will lose weight and enjoy better health by following my diet. It's difficult to predict just how much any one person will benefit, however. Some people who have gone on the Low-Fructose Diet have lost 20 pounds or more and experienced dramatic reductions in blood pressure, blood glucose, and other metabolic measures. But the amount of weight you lose and how much your risk factors for heart disease, diabetes, and other conditions improve will depend on many factors, such as your age, gender, and current weight. The way your body responds to a reduced fructose load will also depend on how elevated and active your fructose enzymes are. And of course, your outcome will depend on how closely you follow the diet.

We can get a sense for what kind of protection you might expect from the Low-Fructose Diet by looking at what population studies tell us. We know that fructose raises uric acid levels. Furthermore, studies show that people with the highest uric acid levels—those in the top 20 to 25 percentile of a population—have the most serious health risks. Specifically, these people are:

- Up to two times more likely to develop hypertension

- Up to five times more likely to die from cardiovascular disease

- Up to three times more likely to develop type 2 diabetes

- 60 percent more likely to have a stroke and

- 3 to 10 times more likely to develop kidney disease

According to some studies, every 1 mg/dl rise in uric acid level has the same relative effect on your health as:

- Adding 10 pounds of body fat

- A 46 mg/dl increase in cholesterol and

- A 10-mm Hg rise in blood pressure

We can't necessarily look at these numbers in reverse—that is, we can't assume that cutting your uric acid level from 8 mg/dl to 7 mg/dl will provide the same protection as reducing your cholesterol by precisely 46 mg/dl, for example. But with these data, we can safely predict that achieving and maintaining healthy uric acid levels by following the Low-Fructose Diet will provide important protection against disease. (I recommend goals of 5.5 mg/dl for men and 5.0 mg/dl for women.)

Here's another way to think about the gains—and losses—you may experience by following my diet. The Low-Fructose Diet takes you back in time, in a sense, because it reduces your intake of this simple sugar to levels typical of Americans a century ago—when only about 5 percent of the population was obese. I believe that by lowering our collective fructose intake, we can reduce current obesity rates by two-thirds or more.

Other research, notably the clinical studies conducted by University of California nutrition researcher Peter J. Havel, PhD, and his colleagues, offer some other clues about the benefits you might experience. Dr. Havel asked his subjects to follow very high-fructose diets, much like many Americans consume every day. His studies suggest that a voracious consumer of fructose-rich foods who adopts the Low-Fructose Diet could experience improvements in conditions of metabolic syndrome and other disease risk factors in the following ranges.

- 5 to 7 percent drop in abdominal fat

- 10 to 20 percent decrease in insulin resistance

- 30 to 50 percent drop in triglycerides

- 10 to 15 percent drop in LDL cholesterol

Dr. Havel's research also suggests that limiting the fructose in your diet will reduce systemic inflammation, an emerging risk factor for heart disease and other conditions.

It's an exciting time in nutrition research. Our understanding of how sweet foods affect health will undoubtedly evolve in the coming years. In the introduction to this book, I described the burgeoning interest in the relationship between fructose, uric acid, and human health as a revolution. I hope *The Sugar Fix* helps lead the charge in combating—and ultimately defeating—obesity and cardiovascular disease.

APPENDICES

RECIPES FOR THE
LOW-FRUCTOSE DIET

"Low in fructose" does not have to mean "low in flavor," as the following pages attest. Many of these recipes were created by Chris Fennell, executive chef and co-owner of the Northwest Grille in Gainesville, Florida (NWGrille.com). Chris graduated from the Art Institute of Fort Lauderdale in 1994, where he received an award for highest achievement in the field of culinary arts.

If you are currently on the Fructose-Free Phase of the diet, you will need to wait before trying any of these recipes. But once you have moved on to the Low-Fructose Lifestyle, you will find that these dishes fit nicely into your daily menu. Each of the recipes provides no more than 3 grams of fructose per serving—and many are 100 percent fructose free.

APPETIZERS

Chicken Nachos

SERVES 6

Preparation time: 10 minutes • Cooking time: 10 to 15 minutes

2 cans (10 ounces each) chunk white chicken meat, chopped

1 cup medium salsa (or hot salsa, if you prefer)

½ teaspoon ground cumin

2 tablespoons chopped fresh cilantro leaves

1 teaspoon lime juice

1 large bag (12 ounces) corn tortilla chips

1 cup low-fat shredded Cheddar or jack cheese

½ cup sliced fresh jalapeño peppers (or substitute green chile peppers), wear plastic gloves when handling

1 cup shredded iceberg lettuce

1 bunch scallions, chopped

½ cup low-fat sour cream (optional)

1. Preheat the oven to 350°F.

2. Combine the chicken, salsa, cumin, cilantro, and lime juice in a microwave-safe bowl. Mix well, place in a microwave oven, and cook on high for 2 minutes.

3. Line the bottom of a lasagna pan with the tortilla chips. Gently distribute the chicken mixture over the chips.

4. Top with the cheese.

5. Bake for about 10 minutes, or until the cheese has melted.

6. Remove the pan from the oven. Top the chicken mixture with the jalapeños, lettuce, and scallions. Top with the sour cream (if using).

NUTRIENTS (PER SERVING)
325 calories, 25 g protein, 30 g total carbohydrates, 1 g fructose, 12 g fat

Endive "Boats" with Blue Cheese, Walnuts, and Crispy Bacon

SERVES 8

Preparation time: 10 minutes • Cooking time: 5 minutes

4 heads endive
6 strips bacon, chopped
1 cup blue cheese crumbles
½ cup chopped walnuts
1 tablespoon freshly chopped chives
Ground black pepper

1. Wash the endive and cut off the stems. Set aside 8 of the large leaves to use as the "boats."

2. Cook the bacon over medium heat until crispy, stirring often. Drain on paper towels.

3. Combine the blue cheese, walnuts, and chives in a bowl.

4. Spoon 1 tablespoon of the blue cheese mixture onto each endive boat and arrange on a platter. Sprinkle each boat with bacon bits and pepper (to taste) and serve.

NUTRIENTS (PER SERVING)
175 calories, 9 g protein, 10 g total carbohydrates, 0 g fructose, 12 g fat

Shrimp and Spinach Dip with Toasted Pita Points

SERVES 8

Preparation time: 10 minutes • Cooking time: 10 to 15 minutes

¾ pound (12-ounce bag) peeled and cooked medium shrimp

1 pound low-fat cream cheese, softened

½ cup low-fat sour cream

¼ cup Knorr (or other brand) dried vegetable soup mix

⅛ teaspoon ground nutmeg

⅛ teaspoon ground red pepper

⅛ teaspoon Old Bay seasoning

Salt and ground black pepper

1 teaspoon lemon juice

1 package (10 ounces) frozen chopped spinach, defrosted and drained of excess water

4 whole wheat pita pockets, cut into triangles

1. Preheat the oven to 350°F.

2. Chop the shrimp (roughly; do not mince). Place in a mixing bowl with the cream cheese, sour cream, soup mix, nutmeg, red pepper, Old Bay seasoning, salt and black pepper (to taste), and lemon juice. Stir well and then mix in the spinach. Place in a serving dish. The dip can be served cold or heated for 2 minutes in a microwave oven.

3. Toast the pita triangles in the oven until crisp, for about 10 to 15 minutes. Arrange on a platter and serve with the dip.

NUTRIENTS (PER SERVING)
320 calories, 22 g protein, 28 g total carbohydrates, 0.2 g fructose, 14 g fat

Oven-Fried Chicken Wings with Blue Cheese Dip

SERVES 6

Preparation time: 20 minutes • Cooking time: 30 minutes

CHICKEN WINGS

1 cup Bisquick mix

1 cup flour

¼ cup Paul Prudhomme Blackened Redfish Magic seasoning

1 teaspoon ground black pepper

½ teaspoon salt

5 pounds chicken wings

BLUE CHEESE DIP

1 cup low-fat sour cream

½ cup blue cheese crumbles

1 teaspoon ground black pepper

½ teaspoon salt

1 teaspoon olive oil

1 teaspoon red wine vinegar

DIPPING SAUCE

Frank's Hot Sauce, Crystal Hot Sauce, or Tabasco Sauce (optional)

1. *To make the chicken wings:* Preheat the oven to 375°F. Combine the Bisquick, flour, seasoning, pepper, and salt in a zip-top bag and mix. Add the chicken wings, about 1 pound at a time, to the flour mixture and coat thoroughly.

2. Place the chicken wings on a baking sheet lined with foil and bake for 30 minutes, or until done.

3. *To make the dip:* While the chicken cooks, combine the sour cream, blue cheese, pepper, salt, oil, and vinegar in a bowl, mix well, and set aside.

4. When the chicken is cooked, serve with blue cheese dip. If using the hot sauce, serve it on the side.

NOTE: For a restaurant-style dipping sauce, combine equal parts hot sauce with melted butter or margarine and mix well.

NUTRIENTS (PER SERVING)
475 calories, 29 g protein, 28 g total carbohydrates, 0 g fructose, 27 g fat

SALADS AND SOUPS

Northern Bean Soup

Preparation time: 30 minutes • Cooking time: 1½ hours

3 strips bacon, chopped

2 tablespoons olive oil

2 ribs celery, chopped

1 white onion, chopped

2 carrots, peeled and chopped

1 red bell pepper, chopped

½ cup diced tomatoes

1 tablespoon chopped garlic

½ cup chopped smoked ham (be sure it contains no honey, sugar, or HFCS) (optional)

½ teaspoon celery salt

½ teaspoon kosher salt

½ teaspoon ground black pepper

½ teaspoon granulated garlic (or garlic powder)

½ teaspoon onion powder (optional)

2 bay leaves

½ teaspoon dried thyme

3 cans (15.5 ounces each) great northern or navy beans, undrained

1 cup water

1. Brown the bacon in a preheated thick-bottomed soup pot.

2. Add the oil, then the celery, onion, carrots, bell pepper, and tomatoes. Sauté for about 3 minutes, or until the vegetables are tender.

3. Add the chopped garlic, celery salt, kosher salt, black pepper, granulated garlic, onion powder (if using), bay leaves, and thyme, stirring for 1 minute.

4. Add the beans, ham (if using), and water. Simmer on low heat for 1 hour. Stir often. If the soup is too thick, add more water. Season with additional salt and pepper to taste. Remove the bay leaves before serving.

NUTRIENTS (PER SERVING)
375 calories, 23 g protein, 53 g total carbohydrates, 3 g fructose, 9 g fat

Spinach Salad with Blue Cheese, Walnuts, and Raspberry Vinaigrette

SERVES 4

Preparation time: 15 minutes • Cooking time: none

SALAD

4 cups baby spinach, washed and drained

½ cup blue cheese crumbles (you may substitute gorgonzola or feta cheese)

½ cup walnuts (either halved or chopped)

6 baby portobello mushrooms, sliced (optional)

16 cherry tomatoes (optional)

1 medium red onion, sliced (optional)

2 hard-cooked eggs (optional)

1 cup fresh raspberries (optional)

DRESSING

¼ cup sugar-free raspberry preserves

½ teaspoon Dijon mustard

Salt and ground black pepper

2 tablespoons raspberry vinegar (you may substitute champagne vinegar, red wine vinegar, or cider vinegar)

3 ounces olive oil

1. *To make the salad:* Place the spinach in a large bowl and top with the blue cheese and walnuts. Add the mushrooms, tomatoes, onion, eggs, and raspberries (if using).

2. *To make the dressing:* Combine the preserves, mustard, salt and pepper (to taste), and vinegar in a bowl and whisk well. Slowly add the oil and stir. Stir or shake the dressing just before using so the ingredients are well mixed. Serve the dressing on the side or drizzle over the salad just before serving.

NUTRIENTS (PER SERVING)
400 calories, 8 g protein, 17 g total carbohydrates, 2 g fructose, 36 g fat

Tomatoes and Mozzarella with Basil Oil

SERVES 4

Preparation time: 10 minutes • Cooking time: none

2 large tomatoes at room temperature (preferably never refrigerated)

2 fresh mozzarella balls (also known as buffalo mozzarella), about 4 ounces each or ½ pound total

Salt and freshly ground black pepper

1 bunch fresh basil (reserve a leaf or two for garnish), washed and dried

½ teaspoon chopped garlic

½ teaspoon Dijon mustard

2 tablespoons lemon juice

3 ounces olive oil

1. Slice the tomatoes and mozzarella and arrange on a platter. Sprinkle with the salt and pepper to taste.

2. Combine the basil, garlic, mustard, and lemon juice in a blender (food processor or stick blender). Blend, and then slowly pour into the oil. When combined, pour over the tomatoes and mozzarella. Garnish with the reserved basil leaves and serve.

NUTRIENTS (PER SERVING)
350 calories, 10 g protein, 6 g total carbohydrates, 1.5 g fructose, 32 g fat

PASTA, RICE, AND SAUCES

Green Corn Sauce

SERVES 6

Preparation time: 10 minutes • Cooking time: 15 to 20 minutes

> 8 cups frozen white corn
>
> 3 tablespoons olive oil
>
> 1 teaspoon hot chile oil (optional)
>
> 1 medium white onion, chopped
>
> 2 teaspoons minced garlic
>
> 1 bunch (about 4 ounces) fresh cilantro leaves, stripped from stems (you should end up with about 1 cup)
>
> 1 cup water
>
> Salt

1. Thaw the frozen corn by soaking it in warm water for 5 to 10 minutes. Drain.

2. Warm the olive oil (and chile oil, if using) in a medium pot over high heat. Add the onion and garlic. Cook the onion quickly, until translucent, for about 3 minutes. Remove the pot from the heat and allow it to cool briefly.

3. Transfer the onion mixture to a blender. Add the cilantro, half of the corn, and ½ cup of the water. Blend at high speed for approximately 1 to 2 minutes or until the sauce is finely pureed.

4. Transfer the sauce back to the pot. Blend the remaining corn with the remaining ½ cup of water. Add the blended corn to the pot and bring to a boil over high heat. Reduce the heat to medium and cook for a total of about 15 minutes, stirring frequently.

5. Add salt to taste. This dish is best served on white rice.

NUTRIENTS (PER SERVING)
260 calories, 6 g protein, 40 g total carbohydrates, 0.2 g fructose, 8 g fat

Spinach Pesto Sauce

SERVES 4

Preparation time: 15 minutes • Cooking time: 10 minutes

2 tablespoons olive oil
½ large white onion, sliced
1 teaspoon minced garlic
1 ounce (by weight) fresh basil, washed and dried
1 bag (10 ounces) fresh baby spinach
¾ cup low-fat evaporated milk
1 cup feta cheese, crumbled
Salt

1. Warm the olive oil over medium heat in a large skillet.

2. Add the onion and garlic. Cook until the onion is translucent.

3. While the onion cooks, add the basil and spinach a few leaves at a time. As the spinach softens and reduces in size, you will be able to add the entire bag. Continue cooking until the spinach and basil leaves have completely softened, about 4 to 5 minutes.

4. Place the spinach mixture, milk, and feta cheese in a blender. Blend at high speed for 1 to 2 minutes, or until mixture has turned into a creamy sauce.

5. Add the salt to taste. This dish is best served with pasta.

NUTRIENTS (PER SERVING)
280 calories, 19 g protein, 11 g total carbohydrates, 0.5 g fructose, 20 g fat

Marvelous and Meatless

SERVES 8

Preparation time: 25 minutes • Cooking time: 40 minutes

8 ounces egg noodles

½ cup chopped yellow onion (or more)

½ cup chopped celery (or more)

½ cup chopped green bell pepper (or more)

1 tablespoon olive oil

½ cup coarsely chopped black olives

1½ teaspoons salt

¼ teaspoon ground black pepper

1 can (10.5 ounces) cream of celery soup

1½ cups cottage cheese (1% fat)

½ cup sour cream

1 cup shredded Cheddar cheese

3 eggs, beaten (optional)

1. Cook the noodles according to package instructions. Drain.

2. Sauté the onion, celery, and bell pepper in the oil in a medium skillet until crisp-tender—about 5 minutes at most (don't overcook).

3. Stir in the olives, salt, and pepper.

4. Combine the soup, cottage cheese, and sour cream in a large bowl.

5. Preheat the oven to 350°F. Coat the inside of a 2-quart baking dish with cooking spray. Arrange one-third of the noodles on the bottom of the dish. Top with half of the vegetables and half of the soup mixture, spreading evenly. Repeat with another one-third of the noodles and the remainder of the vegetables and soup mixture, and then place the final one-third of the noodles on top.

6. Sprinkle the cheese over the top. Pour the eggs (if using) over the cheese. Bake in the oven for 40 minutes.

NUTRIENTS (PER SERVING)
450 calories (with eggs), 21 g protein, 38 g total carbohydrates, 1 g fructose, 23 g fat

Bowtie Pasta Salad

SERVES 8

Preparation time: 20 minutes • Cooking time: 20 minutes

2 boneless, skinless chicken breasts, about
6 ounces each (or precooked frozen chicken)

1 pound dried bowtie pasta

½ teaspoon + 3 ounces olive oil

1 red bell pepper, sliced into strips

¼ cup toasted unsalted pine nuts

1 bunch scallions, chopped

6 cherry tomatoes, halved

½ cup pitted black kalamata olives

2 tablespoons chopped fresh tarragon or
½ teaspoon dried

½ teaspoon chopped garlic

2 tablespoons lemon juice

1 teaspoon Dijon mustard

Salt and ground black pepper

½ cup shredded Parmesan cheese

1. Preheat the oven to 350°F. Bake the chicken breasts for
   20 minutes. Cut into strips. (Or use precooked frozen
   chicken breasts, thawed.)

2. Boil the pasta in salted water according to the package
   directions. Drain and rinse with cold water. Toss with
   ½ teaspoon oil and transfer to a mixing bowl. Add the
   bell pepper, pine nuts, scallions, tomatoes, olives, and
   chicken. Mix well.

3. To make the dressing, combine the tarragon, garlic, lemon juice, 3 ounces olive oil, mustard, and salt and pepper (to taste) in a mixing bowl and whisk. Pour over the pasta salad and mix.

4. Garnish with the cheese and serve.

NUTRIENTS (PER SERVING)
500 calories, 25 g protein, 50 g total carbohydrates, 1 g fructose, 24 g fat

Neapolitan Casserole

SERVES 8

Preparation time: 30 minutes • Cooking time: 50 minutes

1½ pounds ground chuck

1 tablespoon olive oil

1 large yellow onion, chopped

3 cloves garlic, chopped

1 cup coarsely chopped celery

1 cup peeled and chopped carrots

6 ounces canned whole mushrooms, drained

½ cup dry sherry

6 ounces tomato paste

1 can (14.5 ounces) Italian tomatoes, drained

1 tablespoon salt

½ teaspoon ground black pepper

½ teaspoon dried oregano

½ teaspoon dried basil

8 ounces small pasta shells
(equivalent to 2 cups)

10 ounces chopped frozen spinach, defrosted and drained

1 cup grated Cheddar cheese

1 tablespoon grated Parmesan cheese

1. Brown the beef in a large skillet over medium heat with the olive oil. Add the onion, garlic, celery, and carrots and cook for 5 minutes. Add the mushrooms, sherry, tomato paste, tomatoes, salt, pepper, oregano, and basil. Reduce the heat to low and cook for 10 to 15 minutes longer.

2. Cook the pasta shells according to the package directions. When cooked, drain the shells in a colander. Add the spinach.

3. Preheat the oven to 350°F. Mix all ingredients except the cheeses in a large greased baking dish. Top with the Cheddar. Bake in the oven for 30 minutes, or until bubbly. Remove from the oven, sprinkle with the Parmesan, and serve.

NUTRIENTS (PER SERVING)
335 calories, 27 g protein, 37 g total carbohydrates, 3 g fructose, 9 g fat

MAIN DISHES

Ginger Salmon

SERVES 6

Preparation time: 10 minutes • Marinating time: 3 hours
• Cooking time: 25 to 30 minutes

2 tablespoons yellow (or Chinese) mustard
¼ cup soy sauce
1 teaspoon ground fresh ginger
6 salmon fillets (about 6 ounces each)
Lime, cut in wedges

1. To make the marinade, combine the mustard, soy sauce, and ginger in a bowl and whisk.

2. Place the salmon fillets in a baking dish. Pour the marinade over the fillets, turning them to coat both sides.

3. Cover the baking dish with foil and marinate in the refrigerator for at least 3 hours.

4. Bake, covered, at 350°F for 20 minutes. Uncover and cook for an additional 5 minutes, or until done. Serve with the lime wedges.

NUTRIENTS (PER SERVING)
210 calories, 35 g protein, 2 g total carbohydrates, 0 g fructose, 6 g fat

Blackened Tilapia with Scallion Sour Cream and Spiced Pecans

SERVES 4

Preparation time: 30 minutes • Cooking time: 20 to 30 minutes

SPICED PECANS

1 cup pecan halves

1 tablespoon olive oil

1 tablespoon blackening seasoning (use Paul Prudhomme Blackened Redfish Magic or other premixed blackening seasoning; avoid cheaper mixes because they tend to be saltier)

SCALLION SOUR CREAM

1 cup sour cream, preferably low fat

1 bunch scallions, washed and chopped

Pinch of salt

Ground black pepper

Juice of ½ lemon (cut the other half into wedges)

TILAPIA

4 boneless, skinless tilapia fillets (6 to 8 ounces each, see note)

2 tablespoons olive oil

Blackening seasoning (enough to coat the fish on both sides)

2 ounces butter

1. *To make the pecans:* Preheat the oven to 350°F. Toss the pecans in the olive oil and dust with the blackening seasoning. Bake on a baking sheet for 10 to 15 minutes. Remove from the oven and set aside to cool.

2. *To make the sour cream:* Combine the sour cream, scallions, salt, pepper (to taste), and lemon juice. Mix well and refrigerate.

3. *To make the tilapia:* Place the tilapia on a baking pan and coat with the olive oil. Dust liberally on both sides with blackening seasoning.

4. Preheat a large heavy-bottomed skillet on an outdoor grill (on the side burner, if available). Use a cast-iron skillet if possible; a thicker pan retains heat better, resulting in better searing. Do not use nonstick pans due to the high heat required. Outdoor grills are preferred, since the fish will smoke. If you cook this dish inside, place the vent on high.

5. When the pan is heated to medium-high, add the butter. When the butter melts, carefully place the fish in the pan. (Note: Hold the fish at one end, lower it into the pan, and lay it down *away from you* to reduce splashing.)

6. Sear for about 3 minutes, turn the fish, and sear for another 3 minutes. Seared fish should appear dark but not be scorched. If fish begins to scorch, turn it sooner and reduce the heat.

7. Check the fish to make sure its center is thoroughly cooked; it should be white throughout. If it is not done, place the fish on a baking sheet and bake at 350°F for about 10 minutes. When done, top the fish with the sour cream mix, sprinkle with the pecans, and garnish with the lemon wedges.

NOTE: You may use other firm fish such as mahi mahi, grouper, snapper, salmon, or swordfish. Thin fillets are best; thicker fillets may take too long to cook in the middle.

NUTRIENTS (PER SERVING)
525 calories, 39 g protein, 9 g total carbohydrates, 1 g fructose, 39 g fat

Almond-Crusted Mahi Mahi with Lemon Pepper Watercress Salad Topping

SERVES 4

Preparation time: 30 minutes • Cooking time: 20 minutes

CRUST

1 cup sliced almonds (you may substitute pecans, walnuts, or cashews)

1 cup dried bread crumbs (Japanese bread crumbs are best, but plain nonseasoned bread crumbs are fine)

Dash of salt

Ground black pepper

FISH

3 eggs

3 ounces low-fat milk

4 boneless, skinless mahi mahi fillets, 6 to 8 ounces each (you may substitute other fish or even boneless, skinless chicken breasts)

Salt and ground black pepper

½ cup flour

4 ounces olive or vegetable oil

SALAD

Juice of 2 lemons (about 6 tablespoons)

½ teaspoon Dijon mustard

Salt and ground black pepper

¼ cup olive oil

4 ounces watercress, washed and dried (you may substitute spinach, arugula, baby greens, or any spring mix)

½ red onion, finely sliced

1. *To make the crust:* Pulse the almonds in a food processor until they are chopped fine. (Do not overprocess, or the

almonds will gum up. If this happens, add some of the bread crumbs and pulse a little more.) Mix the ground almonds with the bread crumbs and season to taste with the salt and pepper. Set aside.

2. *To make the fish:* Make an egg wash by beating the eggs, then combining them with the milk in a Tupperware (or similar) container large enough to hold 1 fillet of fish.

3. Season the fillets with salt and pepper to taste, dredge them in the flour, and then dip them in the egg wash. Next, press the fish into the almond breading. Make sure the fish is coated completely with the egg wash. Set aside until ready to cook. Do not stack the fish, or they will stick to each other.

4. Warm a large skillet over medium heat. (Do not overheat the skillet, or the almonds will burn.) Cook the fish in the oil. Do not submerge the fish. The breading will absorb the oil, so make sure the pan does not become dry. Sauté both sides for 3 to 5 minutes. Check the center of the fish. If it is not done (the center should be white, not pink), bake in an oven at 350°F for 5 to 10 minutes. The almond crust should be golden brown when done.

5. When the fish is done, remove it from the pan and place it on a plate lined with paper towels to absorb the extra oil.

6. *To make the salad:* Combine the lemon juice, mustard, and salt and pepper (to taste) in a bowl. Whisk while drizzling in the olive oil. Toss the greens, onion, and dressing. Top the fish with the salad mixture and serve.

NUTRIENTS (PER SERVING)
435 calories, 53 g protein, 25 g total carbohydrates, 0.4 g fructose, 13 g fat

Baked Flounder with Lemon Caper Beurre Blanc (White Butter) Sauce

SERVES 4

Preparation time: 15 minutes • Cooking time: 20 minutes

4 boneless, skinless flounder fillets, 6 to 8 ounces each (or other white-fleshed fish such as grouper, sole, or snapper)

1 cup white wine, preferably dry

Salt and pepper (preferably ground white pepper)

6 tablespoons unsalted butter (3 ounces, or about ¾ stick; do not use margarine)

1 shallot, chopped

3 tablespoons drained small capers (nonpareils work best)

Juice of 1 lemon

Parsley or fresh dill (1 tablespoon fresh or ½ teaspoon dry) (optional)

1. Preheat the oven to 400°F. Place the fish on a baking sheet lined with foil. Add 4 ounces of the wine to the pan. Season the fish with the salt and pepper, to taste. Cook the fish for 10 to 15 minutes, or until done. (The fish should be moist when done. Do not cook until dry.)

2. Just before the fish is done, warm a small saucepan over medium heat. Add 2 tablespoons of the butter and sauté the shallot until translucent. The shallot will cook very quickly, so be careful not to burn it.

3. Add the capers and cook. Deglaze the saucepan with the remaining wine and add the lemon juice. Season with more salt and pepper and reduce the liquid to one-third of its original volume.

4. When the liquid is reduced, remove from the heat, whisk in the remaining butter, and add the parsley or dill (if using). Whisk well. The butter should be whisked rapidly to give the sauce a rich, velvety texture. Do not heat the sauce further, or it will separate and become oily.

5. Pour the sauce over the baked fish and serve immediately.

NUTRIENTS (PER SERVING)
360 calories, 34 g protein, 8 g total carbohydrates, 1 g fructose, 19 g fat

Sesame-Crusted Yellowfin Tuna

SERVES 4

Preparation time: 15 minutes • Cooking time: 5 minutes

TUNA

4 yellowfin tuna steaks, about 6 ounces each
(at least 1" thick)

4 tablespoons rice wine vinegar

½ cup flour

4 tablespoons cornstarch

2 tablespoons sesame seeds

2 tablespoons black sesame seeds

¼ cup canola oil

WASABI SOY VINAIGRETTE

1½ teaspoons to 1 tablespoon wasabi paste

2 tablespoons soy sauce

2 tablespoons rice wine vinegar

½ teaspoon chopped garlic

¼ teaspoon ground ginger

4 tablespoons orange juice

¼ cup canola oil

½ cup chopped scallions

1. *To make the tuna:* Moisten the tuna steaks with the 4 tablespoons vinegar. Combine the flour, cornstarch, and sesame seeds in a bowl, then press the tuna into this mixture, coating all sides. Place the tuna steaks on a plate.

2. Warm a large skillet over medium-high heat. Add the ¼ cup oil and heat for 30 seconds. Carefully place the tuna steaks in the pan and sear for 2 minutes on each side until golden brown.

3. *To make the vinaigrette:* Combine the wasabi paste, soy
   sauce, the 2 tablespoons vinegar, garlic, ginger, and orange
   juice in a bowl, then whisk while slowly drizzling in the oil.
   Add the scallions and serve with the tuna steaks in small
   bowls on the side.

NUTRIENTS (PER SERVING)
600 calories, 58 g protein, 35 g total carbohydrates, 0.5 g fructose, 24 g fat

Grilled Salmon with Cucumber Dill Relish

SERVES 4

Preparation time: 15 minutes • Cooking time: 15 minutes

CUCUMBER DILL RELISH
1 seedless European cucumber, chopped
1 small red onion, chopped
1 tablespoon chopped fresh dill
2 tablespoons rice wine vinegar
1 teaspoon olive oil
Salt and ground black pepper
⅛ teaspoon ground red pepper
Lemon wedges (optional)

SALMON
4 salmon fillets (about 6 ounces each)
2 tablespoons olive oil
Salt and ground black pepper

1. *To make the relish:* Combine the cucumber, onion, dill, vinegar, 1 teaspoon oil, salt and black pepper (to taste), and red pepper in a bowl, mix, and set aside. The relish can be prepared in advance.

2. *To make the salmon:* Preheat the grill. Rub the salmon with the 2 tablespoons oil and sprinkle with salt and pepper, to taste. Grill over medium-high heat until cooked, about 6 minutes per side. You can also cook the fish in an oven at 350°F for 12 to 16 minutes without turning.

3. Top the salmon with the relish and serve. Garnish with the lemon wedges, if using.

NUTRIENTS (PER SERVING)
300 calories, 35 g protein, 4 g total carbohydrates, 1 g fructose, 14 g fat

Roasted Chicken Breasts with Tomato Lime BBQ Glaze

SERVES 4

Preparation time: 20 minutes • Cooking time: 60 minutes

1 teaspoon + 2 tablespoons olive oil

1 small white onion, chopped

1 teaspoon chopped garlic

½ teaspoon red-pepper flakes

¼ teaspoon ground cumin

¼ teaspoon ground black pepper

2 cups chopped tomatoes

3 tablespoons soy sauce

2 tablespoons lime juice

1½ tablespoons Splenda (white granulated)

4 chicken breasts, bone in

Salt and ground black pepper

1. To make the glaze, warm 1 teaspoon of the oil in a saucepan over medium-high heat. Sauté the onion until translucent. Add the garlic, red-pepper flakes, cumin, black pepper, and tomatoes. Cook for 5 minutes. Add the soy sauce, lime juice, and Splenda, and cook for 5 minutes longer.

2. Remove from the heat and allow to cool. Spoon the mixture into a blender or food processor and puree.

3. Preheat the oven to 375°F. Line a baking sheet with foil. Place the chicken breasts on the sheet and drizzle with 2 tablespoons of the olive oil. Season with salt and pepper, to taste. Place in the oven.

4. After 30 minutes, begin basting with the glaze. Cook for 20 to 30 minutes longer, until the chicken is done, basting several times. You can serve the leftover glaze on the side or drizzle it over the chicken when it's done.

NUTRIENTS (PER SERVING)
250 calories, 30 g protein, 10 g total carbohydrates, 2 g fructose, 10 g fat

Grilled Chicken Breasts over Orzo Pasta with Artichoke Hearts and Feta Cheese

SERVES 4

Preparation time: 20 minutes • Cooking time: 25 minutes

8 ounces dry orzo pasta

3 tablespoons olive oil

4 boneless, skinless chicken breasts (4 to 6 ounces each)

Salt and ground black pepper

1 teaspoon chopped garlic

1 jar (8 ounces) quartered artichoke hearts, drained

Sliced mushrooms (optional)

Sun-dried tomatoes (optional)

Juice of 1 lemon

1 teaspoon chopped fresh thyme

½ cup feta cheese crumbles (reduced fat preferable; may substitute other cheeses, such as shredded Italian cheese blends or shredded Parmesan)

1 lemon, cut into wedges

1. Boil the orzo in a large pot of salted water according to the package instructions. Stir frequently to prevent the orzo from sticking to the bottom of the pan. Drain and rinse with cold water. Toss with 1 teaspoon of the oil and set aside. (You can prepare the pasta in advance and store it in the refrigerator.)

2. Preheat the grill. Place the chicken breasts on a plate and drizzle with 2 teaspoons of the oil. Season with the salt and pepper to taste (use only a little salt because feta cheese is salty). Grill the chicken for 7 to 10 minutes per side, or until done. Or bake it in an oven at 350°F for about 30 minutes. When the chicken is done, cut it into strips and set it aside. (You can prepare the chicken in advance and store it in the refrigerator.)

3. Warm the remaining 2 tablespoons of the oil in a large skillet over medium heat.

4. Place the chicken breast strips in the skillet and toss them in the olive oil. Add the garlic and sauté for 2 minutes. Do not burn the garlic.

5. Add the artichoke hearts and the mushrooms and tomatoes (if using) and cook for 2 to 3 minutes over medium heat.

6. Toss in the orzo and mix well. Stir in the lemon juice and thyme.

7. When the pasta is hot, add the feta cheese. Serve when the cheese has melted.

8. Garnish with the lemon wedges.

NUTRIENTS (PER SERVING)
500 calories, 51 g protein, 48 g total carbohydrates, 0 g fructose, 11 g fat

Tortilla-Crusted Chicken Breasts with Black Bean Salsa

SERVES 4

Preparation time: 20 minutes • Cooking time: 20 to 30 minutes

BLACK BEAN SALSA

1 can (15 ounces) cooked black beans, drained (and rinsed, if you like)

1 jalapeño pepper, finely chopped (wear plastic gloves when handling)

1 small white onion, chopped

½ teaspoon chopped garlic

1 small green or yellow bell pepper, chopped

1 tablespoon chopped fresh cilantro

1 teaspoon olive oil

1 teaspoon lime or lemon juice

Salt and ground black pepper

CHICKEN BREASTS

2 cups tortilla chips, crushed in a food processor (preferably red, blue, or other colors)

¾ cup plain dried bread crumbs

¼ teaspoon ground cumin

1 egg

½ cup low-fat milk

4 boneless, skinless chicken breasts, 4 to 6 ounces each (or substitute fish, such as grouper, mahi mahi, or tilapia)

Salt and ground black pepper

½ cup flour

1. *To make the salsa:* Combine the beans, jalapeño pepper, onion, garlic, bell pepper, cilantro, oil, juice, and salt and pepper (to taste) in a mixing bowl and refrigerate until ready to serve. You can prepare the salsa in advance.

2. *To make the chicken:* Combine the tortilla chips, bread crumbs, and cumin. Spread the mixture onto a large plate.

3. Make an egg wash by whisking the egg and milk in a Tupperware (or similar) container.

4. Preheat the oven to 375°F. Season the chicken with the salt and pepper, to taste. Coat a chicken breast in the flour on both sides and dip in the egg wash. Make sure the chicken is coated completely with the egg wash. Next, press it into the tortilla mixture and place it on a foil-lined baking sheet. Repeat with other chicken breasts and bake for 20 to 30 minutes. (Oven temperatures vary, so check to make sure it is done.)

5. Top the chicken with the salsa and serve.

NUTRIENTS (PER SERVING)
350 calories, 36 g protein, 40 g total carbohydrates, 0 g fructose, 6 g fat

Barbecued Chicken, Chinese Style

SERVES 4

Preparation time: 30 minutes to 2 hours
• Cooking time: 50 to 60 minutes

1 teaspoon dry mustard
½ teaspoon ground ginger
¼ teaspoon ground black pepper
½ teaspoon garlic powder
⅓ cup soy sauce
3 tablespoons canola oil
1 frying chicken, about 2½ pounds, cut into quarters

1. To make the marinade, mix the mustard, ginger, pepper, and garlic powder together, and then add the soy sauce and oil.

2. Place the chicken in a large Tupperware (or similar) container. Brush with the marinade, completely coating each piece. Place the chicken in the refrigerator. Marinate for at least 30 minutes, and up to 10 hours or more for greater flavor, periodically brushing more marinade onto the chicken.

3. Place the chicken on a shallow oven pan and bake at 350°F for 50 minutes, or until tender. Brush the chicken with the pan drippings or with additional marinade every 15 minutes or so. The chicken will be brown and crisp when it is done.

NUTRIENTS (PER SERVING)
355 calories, 23 g protein, 3 g total carbohydrates, 0 g fructose, 28 g fat

Lime Tarragon Chicken

SERVES 6

Preparation time: 2 hours or more, largely unattended
• Cooking time: 30 to 40 minutes

**6 boneless, skinless chicken breasts
(6 ounces each)**

½ cup olive oil

½ cup lime juice (about 4 fresh limes)

1 tablespoon chopped onion

2 teaspoons dried tarragon

1¼ teaspoons salt

⅛ teaspoon ground black pepper

½ teaspoon Tabasco sauce

1. Place the chicken in a baking dish.

2. Combine the oil, lime juice, onion, tarragon, salt, pepper, and Tabasco sauce in a bowl and mix to make a sauce.

3. Brush the sauce over the chicken. Pour any extra sauce over the chicken.

4. Cover and marinate in the refrigerator for 2 to 4 hours.

5. Preheat the broiler. Place the chicken on the broiler rack or in a shallow pan and broil for about 10 minutes, until the chicken has browned. Switch the oven to "bake" and cook at 350°F for an additional 20 to 30 minutes, turning the chicken occasionally.

NUTRIENTS (PER SERVING)
310 calories, 28 g protein, 2 g total carbohydrates, 0.2 g fructose, 20 g fat

Puckering Beef

SERVES 4

Preparation time: 10 to 15 minutes • Cooking time: 20 minutes

2 teaspoons garlic salt

⅛ teaspoon ground black pepper

Pinch of ground cumin

1½ pounds beef round, chopped into bite-size cubes

3 tablespoons olive oil

1 medium red onion, sliced

½ teaspoon ground paprika

1 teaspoon hot chile oil

2 large tomatoes, chopped into small pieces

⅓ cup white vinegar

2 tablespoons soy sauce

Tabasco sauce (optional)

1. Combine the garlic salt, pepper, and cumin in a small bowl. Season the beef with the garlic mixture and set aside.

2. Warm the olive oil in a medium-size pot for several minutes over high heat. Add the onion and reduce the heat to medium-high until the onion is translucent, about 2 to 3 minutes. Add the paprika and chile oil.

3. Reduce the heat to medium and add the beef to the pot, stirring frequently. Cook until the beef has lightly browned, about 3 minutes.

4. Add the tomatoes and increase the temperature to high. Then add the vinegar and soy sauce. Bring the pot to a boil, and cook over high heat for 5 minutes. As the vinegar boils, some of the liquid will reduce.

5. Remove the pot from the heat and let it cool slightly for 3 to
    5 minutes. This dish is best served with white rice. You may
    add Tabasco sauce, to taste.

NUTRIENTS (PER SERVING)
375 calories, 39 g protein, 8 g total carbohydrates, 2 g fructose, 20 g fat

Grilled New York Strip Steak with Portobello Mushrooms and Garlic Butter

SERVES 4

Preparation time: 15 minutes • Cooking time: 20 to 25 minutes

4 New York strip steaks, 6 to 8 ounces each, though any good-quality cut of beef—such as tenderloin (filet mignon), rib-eye (Delmonico), or top sirloin—will do. (Bottom round sirloin and similar cuts are not recommended, however.)

4 medium portobello mushroom caps (one for each steak)

Olive oil

Salt and ground black pepper

Granulated garlic or garlic powder

1 teaspoon fresh chopped thyme, or ½ teaspoon dried

1 teaspoon chopped garlic

1 tablespoon chopped parsley

3 ounces unsalted butter (about ¾ stick), softened

1. Place the steaks and mushrooms on a baking sheet and coat with the oil. (The mushrooms absorb a lot of oil, so be generous.) Season with salt, pepper, and granulated garlic to taste. Add the thyme, if using. Set aside.

2. To make the garlic butter, blend the chopped garlic and parsley with the softened (important—*not* melted) butter. Add salt and pepper to taste.

3. Preheat the grill to medium-high. When the grill is hot, cook the mushrooms, cap side down, for 5 minutes, then turn them over and move to a cooler part of the grill. Then cook the steaks to your liking.

4. When the steaks are done, place each one on top of a grilled mushroom, then top the steak with the garlic butter.

NUTRIENTS (PER 6-OUNCE SERVING)
630 calories, 38 g protein, 5 g total carbohydrates, 0 g fructose, 50 g fat

London Broil with Caramelized Onions

SERVES 4

Preparation time: 30 minutes • Marinating time: 1 hour
• Cooking time: 30 to 40 minutes

2 tablespoons butter
2 red onions, thinly sliced
4 tablespoons red wine vinegar
1 flank steak, 1½ to 2 pounds
1 tablespoon olive oil
Salt and ground black pepper
1 teaspoon granulated garlic or garlic powder
1 teaspoon dried rosemary

1. Melt the butter in a heavy-bottomed soup pan over low to medium heat. Add the onions and cook for about 20 minutes, stirring frequently to prevent scorching. If the onions begin to burn, reduce the heat to low and continue stirring. When the onions start to brown, pour in the vinegar and cook for 2 minutes.

2. Place the flank steak in a lasagna pan and rub with the oil. Sprinkle with the salt and pepper to taste, the garlic, and rosemary. Refrigerate for 1 hour.

3. Remove the lasagna pan from the refrigerator and bring the steak to room temperature by allowing it to sit on the counter for 20 minutes before cooking. Turn on the oven's broiler and place the rack on the lowest level.

4. Place the lasagna pan in the oven and cook the steak for 15 minutes for medium-rare, longer if desired.

5. When cooked, remove the lasagna pan from the oven and let the steak sit for 5 minutes. Place the steak on a cutting board and slice against the grain. Serve topped with the caramelized onions.

NUTRIENTS (PER SERVING)
430 calories, 50 g protein, 6 g total carbohydrates, 1 g fructose, 20 g fat

Portobello Mushroom "Burgers"

SERVES 4

Preparation time: 60 minutes • Cooking time: 10 to 15 minutes

- 4 large portobello mushroom caps (no stems)
- ½ cup olive oil
- 1 teaspoon chopped garlic
- 1 teaspoon soy sauce
- 1 teaspoon chopped fresh thyme or ½ teaspoon dried thyme
- 1 teaspoon Dijon mustard
- ½ teaspoon lemon juice
- Salt and ground black pepper
- 4 whole grain buns
- Cheese, sliced tomatoes, sliced onions, or alfalfa sprouts (optional)

1. Place the portobello caps in a large mixing bowl. Combine the oil, garlic, soy sauce, thyme, mustard, and lemon juice in a small bowl and mix. Pour this mixture over the mushrooms and add salt and pepper to taste. Toss the mushroom caps until coated. Marinate for 1 hour.

2. Preheat the grill to medium-high. Grill the mushrooms, cap side down, for about 5 minutes, then turn and cook them for 5 minutes longer.

3. Place the mushrooms on the buns, and top with your choice of cheese, tomatoes, onions, or alfalfa sprouts (if using).

NUTRIENTS (PER SERVING)
400 calories, 6 g protein, 28 g total carbohydrates, 1 g fructose, 31 g fat

DESSERTS

Sugar-Free Vanilla Ice Cream with Bananas in Rum Butter Sauce

SERVES 4

Preparation time: 5 minutes • Cooking time: 5 minutes

2 cubes butter (about 1 ounce each)

2 bananas, cut into thick slices

4 tablespoons rum (you may substitute brandy or bourbon)

Dash of vanilla extract

¼ teaspoon Splenda (brown sugar style)

Pinch of salt

4 scoops (2 cups) sugar-free vanilla ice cream or frozen yogurt

1. Melt 1 cube of the butter in a small saucepan over medium heat. Sauté the banana slices quickly. Do not stir them too much, or the bananas will get mushy. Remove from the heat. Add the rum, vanilla extract, Splenda, and salt.

2. Return the pan to the heat. Be careful, because the pan will flame up briefly as the rum burns off. Cook for 1 to 2 minutes, and then stir in the second butter cube. When the butter melts, pour the sauce over the ice cream and serve.

NUTRIENTS (PER SERVING)
285 calories, 3 g protein, 29 g total carbohydrates, 4 g fructose, 16 g fat

Sugar-Free New York Style Cheesecake

SERVES 12

Preparation time: 30 minutes • Cooking time: 90 minutes for cheesecake, 10 minutes for crust

CRUST

1 box (5.5 ounces) sugar-free vanilla wafers (such as Murray)

2 tablespoons butter, melted

2 tablespoons flour

FILLING

5 blocks cream cheese (8 ounces each, 2½ pounds total), softened

1 cup Splenda (white granulated)

2 tablespoons sour cream

Dash of salt

1 teaspoon vanilla extract

2 tablespoons cornstarch

1 lemon, juiced and peeled

4 whole eggs

2 egg yolks

1. *To make the crust:* Blend the vanilla wafers in a food processor with the melted butter until smooth.

2. Preheat the oven to 325°F. Coat the inside of a 10" × 3" springform pan with cooking spray and dust with the flour. Wrap the outside bottom of the pan in foil and line the interior with waxed paper.

3. Press the crust mixture into the bottom of the pan and bake for 10 minutes. Remove from the oven and set aside.

4. *To make the filling:* Combine the cream cheese, Splenda, sour cream, salt, vanilla extract, and cornstarch in a stand mixer with a paddle. Mix on low speed for 5 minutes. Scrape

down the sides of the bowl and the paddle with a spatula and mix for 1 minute longer. (You can also use a hand mixer on low speed.)

5. Add the lemon juice and the lemon peel to the mixture. (Be sure to strain out any seeds before adding.)

6. Crack the eggs and add them to the yolks in a mixing cup. Do not whisk. Slowly add the eggs into the cream cheese mixture while blending on low speed. When fully combined, stop the mixer and scrape down the sides and paddle again. Return to low speed and mix for 10 minutes longer.

7. Check that the oven is still at 325°F. Pour the batter onto the prebaked crust. Place the foil-wrapped pan onto a jelly roll pan (or 12" cake pan) with $\frac{1}{4}$" of water in the pan. (The water will help the cheesecake bake without cracking.)

8. Carefully place the pan in the oven and bake for about $1\frac{1}{2}$ hours. Check often; if the cheesecake rises quickly and the center is loose, turn down the oven temperature to 275°F and continue baking. The cheesecake is done when the center of the cake is firm when you jiggle the pan.

9. When the cheesecake is done, remove the springform pan from the jelly roll pan and allow it to cool on the counter. (Leave the jelly roll pan in the oven until it cools so you don't spill hot water when you remove it from the oven.)

10. When the cheesecake is cool, cover it in plastic wrap and refrigerate overnight. Carefully remove the cake from the springform pan and serve. (Tip: Use a slicing knife to cut the cake. Rinse the blade in hot water and wipe clean between each slice.)

NOTE: Cheesecake freezes well. Covered with plastic wrap and placed in a freezer bag, leftovers will keep for a few months.

NUTRIENTS (PER SERVING)
450 calories, 11 g protein, 17 g total carbohydrates, 0 g fructose, 40 g fat

Rice Pudding

SERVES 8

Preparation time: 3 hours, largely unattended

• Cooking time: 15 minutes

1 cup long-grain rice

2 cups water

1 cinnamon stick (may substitute ¼ teaspoon
ground cinnamon)

4 strips lemon peel

4 cups low-fat milk

Dash of salt

1 can (8 ounces) evaporated low-fat milk

2 cups Splenda (white granulated)

1 tablespoon butter

2 egg yolks, whisked

Ground cinnamon for garnish

1. Place the rice and water in a medium saucepan. Let the rice soak for 3 hours.

2. Add the cinnamon and lemon peel to the same pan. Cook over medium heat until the water evaporates.

3. Add 3½ cups of the milk to the pan with the rice, stirring constantly. Add the salt. Continue stirring and then add the evaporated milk and Splenda. Bring to a boil for about 5 minutes.

4. Warm the remaining ½ cup of the milk in a separate pot over low heat. Mix the butter and egg yolks in a bowl with the warmed milk and whisk rapidly. Then add the mixture to the rice and continue stirring for 5 minutes. Remove from the heat and remove the cinnamon stick and lemon peel.

5. Transfer the pudding to a large bowl. Cover with plastic wrap and let it cool, if you like, or serve it warm. Garnish with the ground cinnamon. If prepared in advance, refrigerate until serving.

NUTRIENTS (PER SERVING)
210 calories, 9 g protein, 35 g total carbohydrates, 0 g fructose, 4 g fat

Warm Strawberry Tart

SERVES 4

Preparation time: 20 minutes • Cooking time: 30 minutes

TOPPING
1 pint strawberries, washed and sliced
2 tablespoons Splenda (white granulated)
½ teaspoon lemon juice
Pinch of salt
1 teaspoon brandy (optional)

CRUST
1 package (5.5 ounces) sugar-free vanilla wafers
2 tablespoons butter, melted

FILLING
8 ounces low-fat cream cheese, softened
½ teaspoon vanilla extract
½ teaspoon lemon juice
Pinch of salt
2 tablespoons Splenda (white granulated)
Cool Whip, sugar free

1. *To make the topping:* Place the strawberries in a bowl and top with the Splenda, lemon juice, salt, and brandy (if using). Set aside and toss occasionally while preparing the crust and filling.

2. *To make the crust:* Preheat the oven to 350°F. Crush the vanilla wafers in a food processor or dough press. Mix the butter into the wafers until doughy. Press this mixture into a 9" pie pan. Bake for 10 minutes.

3. *To make the filling:* Mix the cream cheese, vanilla extract, lemon juice, salt, and Splenda in a bowl. Spread the mixture into the prebaked crust. Bake at 350°F for 15 to 20 minutes. Remove from the oven and spoon the topping over the tart. Serve with the Cool Whip.

NUTRIENTS (PER SERVING)
380 calories, 10 g protein, 40 g total carbohydrates, 2.2 g fructose, 19 g fat

THE FRUCTOSE CONTENT
OF COMMON FOODS

Use the following tables to select foods based on their fructose content. The values listed below represent estimates based on typical serving sizes. In some cases, averages were used because the fructose content of similar foods may vary. (In a few cases where information about a food's fructose content was difficult to determine, we have listed its maximum possible fructose content—"0.5 or less," for example.) Serving sizes are based on typical portions listed on product labels. Foods that contain very small traces of fructose—less than 0.1 gram per serving—are listed as 0 gram. We have not included charts for certain food groups, including meat, fish, and legumes, because most foods in these categories contain little or no fructose. Estimates were made using information provided by the USDA, nutrient analysis software created by ESHA Research, and individual food manufacturers.

The Fructose Content of Fresh and Processed Foods

FRUITS

FRUIT	SERVING SIZE	GRAMS OF FRUCTOSE
Fructose Free/Very Low Fructose		
Limes	1 medium	0
Lemons	1 medium	0.6*

FRUIT	SERVING SIZE	GRAMS OF FRUCTOSE
Cranberries	1 cup	0.7
Passion fruit	1 medium	0.9

Low Fructose

FRUIT	SERVING SIZE	GRAMS OF FRUCTOSE
Prune	1 medium	1.2
Apricot	1 medium	1.3
Guava	2 medium	2.2
Date (Deglet Noor style)	1 medium	2.6
Plum	1 medium	2.6*
Cantaloupe	⅛ of medium melon	2.8
Raspberries	1 cup	3.0*

Moderate Fructose

FRUIT	SERVING SIZE	GRAMS OF FRUCTOSE
Clementine	1 medium	3.4
Kiwifruit	1 medium	3.4*
Blackberries	1 cup	3.5*
Star fruit	1 medium	3.6
Cherries, sweet	10	3.8
Strawberries	1 cup	3.8*
Cherries, sour	1 cup	4.0
Pineapple	1 slice (3½ inches x ¾ inches)	4.0*
Grapefruit, pink or red	½ medium	4.3*
Boysenberries	1 cup	4.6
Tangerine/ mandarin orange	1 medium	4.8*
Nectarine	1 medium	5.4
Peach	1 medium	5.9
Orange (navel)	1 medium	6.1*
Papaya	½ medium	6.3*
Honeydew	⅛ of medium melon	6.7*
Banana	1 medium	7.1
Blueberries	1 cup	7.4
Date (Medjool)	1 medium	7.7

FRUIT	SERVING SIZE	GRAMS OF FRUCTOSE
	High Fructose	
Apple (composite)	1 medium	9.5
Persimmon	1 medium	10.6
Watermelon	1/16 of medium melon	11.3
Pear	1 medium	11.8
Raisins	1/4 cup	12.3
Grapes, seedless (green or red)	1 cup	12.4
Mango	1/2 medium	16.2*
Apricots, dried	1 cup	16.4
Figs, dried	1 cup	23.0

*Good sources of vitamin C are noted with an asterisk. Vitamin C helps counter the effects of fructose.

VEGETABLES

VEGETABLE	SERVING SIZE	GRAMS OF FRUCTOSE
	Fructose Free/Very Low Fructose	
Alfalfa sprouts	1 cup	0
Avocado	1/4 medium	0
Endive	1/2 cup	0
Garlic	3 cloves	0
Lettuce, red leaf (shredded)	1 cup	0
Mushroom, portobello	1 (about 3 ounces)	0
Olives, green, black, or calamata	6 small or 4 large	0
Parsley	2 tablespoons	0
Sauerkraut	1/2 cup	0
Spinach	1 cup	0
Turnip greens, cooked	1/2 cup	0
Watercress	1 sprig	0
Kale	1/2 cup	0.1
Mushrooms, white	1/2 cup	0.1

VEGETABLE	SERVING SIZE	GRAMS OF FRUCTOSE
Mustard greens	½ cup	0.1
Yams	½ cup	0.1
Artichoke	1 medium	0.2
Celery	1 medium rib	0.2
Lettuce, green leaf (shredded)	1 cup	0.2
Radishes	4 medium	0.2
Collards, cooked	½ cup	0.3 or less
Lettuce, butterhead (shredded)	1 cup	0.3
Pickle, dill	1 medium	0.3
Okra	8 (3-inch pods)	0.4
Cauliflower	½ cup	0.5
Leek	1 whole	0.6
Potato, russet	1 medium	0.6
Rhubarb	1 cup	0.6
Green beans (snap beans)	½ cup	0.7
Lettuce, iceberg (shredded)	1 cup	0.7
Squash, yellow	½ cup	0.7
Asparagus	5 medium spears	0.9
Brussels sprouts	5 sprouts	0.9
Cabbage, green	½ cup	0.9
Swiss chard, cooked	½ cup	0.9 or less

Low Fructose

Kohlrabi, chopped	½ cup	1.0
Parsnips	½ cup	1.0
Potato, red	1 medium	1.0
Broccoli	1 stalk	1.1
Carrots, baby	5 medium	1.2
Cabbage, red	1 cup	1.3
Corn, yellow	1 medium ear	1.3

VEGETABLE	SERVING SIZE	GRAMS OF FRUCTOSE
Rutabaga	½ cup	1.3
Green bell pepper	1 medium	1.4
Cucumber, peeled	⅓ medium	1.5
Carrot	1 large	1.7
Tomato	1 medium	1.7
Pumpkin, mashed	½ cup	1.8
Onion, yellow	1 medium	1.9
Zucchini	1 medium	1.9
Beets, sliced	½ cup	2.2
Sweet potato	1 medium	2.6
Eggplant, cubed	1 cup	2.7
Red bell pepper	1 medium	2.7

Moderate Fructose

Pickle, sweet	1 medium	3.1
Peas	1 cup	4.2

BREADS AND GRAINS

GRAIN	SERVING SIZE	GRAMS OF FRUCTOSE

Fructose Free/Very Low Fructose

Bulgur, cooked	1 cup	0
Matzo, plain	1 piece	0
Melba toast, plain	1 slice	0
Pretzels, hard	1 serving (per product label)	0
Saltines	5 crackers	0
Triscuits	7 crackers	0
Barley	1 cup	0.1
Pasta (all varieties)	1 cup	0.1
Rice, white	1 cup	0.1
Tortilla, corn	1 small	0.1
Tortilla, flour	1 large	0.1
Rice, brown	1 cup	0.3
English muffin, sourdough	1 muffin	0.4

GRAIN	SERVING SIZE	GRAMS OF FRUCTOSE
Club Crackers, original	4 crackers	0.5
Ritz Crackers, original	5 crackers	0.6
Biscuits, plain or buttermilk	1 medium	0.6
Pita, white	6-inch round	0.8
Pumpernickel bread	1 slice	0.8
Rye bread	1 slice	0.8
Cornmeal	1 cup	0.9

Low Fructose

Bagel	1 medium	1.0
Egg bread	1 slice	1.0
French bread	1 slice	1.0
Italian bread	1 slice	1.0
White bread	1 slice	1.0
Oat bread	1 slice	1.3
Whole wheat bread	1 slice	1.3
Mixed grain bread	1 slice	1.8
Whole grain bread	1 slice	1.8
Wheat Thins, reduced fat	16 crackers	2.0
Corn bread (from mix)	¼ cup mix	3.0

Moderate Fructose

Raisin bread	1 slice	4.0

BREAD TOPPINGS AND CONDIMENTS

CONDIMENT	SERVING SIZE	GRAMS OF FRUCTOSE

Fructose Free/Very Low Fructose

Mustard (most varieties)	1 teaspoon	0
Peanut butter, chunky, natural style	2 tablespoons	0.5

CONDIMENT	SERVING SIZE	GRAMS OF FRUCTOSE
Peanut butter, chunky	2 tablespoons	0.7

Low Fructose

Honey mustard	1 teaspoon	1.0
Ketchup	1 tablespoon	1.4
Peanut butter, smooth	2 tablespoons	1.4
Barbecue sauce	1 tablespoon	2.5

Moderate Fructose

Jams and jellies	1 tablespoon	5.0[1]

[1] Can be as high as 10 grams per tablespoon

SALAD DRESSINGS

DRESSING	SERVING SIZE	GRAMS OF FRUCTOSE

Fructose Free/Very Low Fructose

Red wine vinegar	2 tablespoons	0
White vinegar	2 tablespoons	0
Caesar dressing	1 tablespoon	0.1
Ranch dressing	1 tablespoon	0.2
Blue cheese dressing	1 tablespoon	0.3
Italian dressing	1 tablespoon	0.5
Cider vinegar	2 tablespoons	0.8

Low Fructose

French dressing	1 tablespoon	1.2
Thousand Island dressing	1 tablespoon	1.2
Coleslaw dressing	1 tablespoon	1.6

Moderate Fructose

Balsamic vinegar	2 tablespoons	2.4

BREAKFAST CEREALS

CEREAL	SERVING SIZE	GRAMS OF FRUCTOSE
Fructose Free/Very Low Fructose		
Cream of Wheat	1 cup	0
Grape-Nuts	½ cup	0
Grits	1 cup	0
Oatmeal, plain instant	1 cup	0
Shredded wheat	1 cup	0
Cheerios, toasted whole grain oat	1 cup	0.5
Low Fructose		
Kellogg's Corn Flakes	1 cup	1.0
Rice Chex	1¼ cups	1.0
Rice Krispies	1¼ cups	1.4
Kix	1¼ cups	1.5
Wheaties	¾ cup	1.9
Special K	1 cup	2.0
Total	¾ cup	2.3
Life	¾ cup	3.0
Moderate Fructose		
Bran flakes	¾ cup	3.5
Honey Bunches of Oats	¾ cup	3.5
Oatmeal Squares	1 cup	4.0
Cinnamon Toast Crunch	¾ cup	4.8
Lucky Charms	¾ cup	5.5
Froot Loops	1 cup	5.9
Cap'n Crunch	¾ cup	6.0
Cocoa Puffs	¾ cup	6.0
Frosted Mini-Wheats	24 biscuits	6.0
Honey-Comb	1½ cups	6.0
Kellogg's Frosted Flakes	¾ cup	6.0

CEREAL	SERVING SIZE	GRAMS OF FRUCTOSE
Granola, without raisins	½ cup	7.0
Raisin bran	1 cup	7.6

High Fructose

Smart Start	1¼ cups	9.5

BEVERAGES

BEVERAGE	SERVING SIZE	GRAMS OF FRUCTOSE

Fructose Free/Very Low Fructose

Coffee	8 ounces	0
Tea, black	8 ounces	0
Tea, herb	8 ounces	0

Moderate Fructose

Tomato juice	8 ounces	4.0
Vegetable juice cocktail	8 ounces	4.0
Carrot juice	8 ounces	4.6
Gatorade	8 ounces	5.6
Grapefruit juice	8 ounces	6.6

High Fructose

Lemonade	8 ounces	10.5
Orange juice	8 ounces	10.7
Cherry drink	8 ounces	11.3
Pineapple juice	8 ounces	11.4
Fruit/vegetable blends	8 ounces	12.4
Cranberry juice cocktail	8 ounces	12.6
Cranberry juice	8 ounces	13.0
Fruit punch	8 ounces	13.8
Cherry juice	8 ounces	14.0
Apple juice	8 ounces	16.0
Ginger ale	12 ounces	17.0
Grape juice (canned)	8 ounces	18.8

BEVERAGE	SERVING SIZE	GRAMS OF FRUCTOSE
Prune juice	8 ounces	20.2
Cola	12 ounces	20.2
Root beer	12 ounces	22.2

ALCOHOLIC BEVERAGES

ALCOHOLIC BEVERAGE	SERVING SIZE	GRAMS OF FRUCTOSE

Fructose Free/Very Low Fructose

Beer[1]	12 ounces	0
Gin	1.5 ounces	0
Rum	1.5 ounces	0
Vodka	1.5 ounces	0
Whiskey	1.5 ounces	0
Vermouth, dry	1 ounce	0.8
Wine, red	5 ounces	0.9 or less
Wine, white	5 ounces	0.9 or less

Low Fructose

Sherry, medium dry	2 ounces	1.1
Wine, rosé	5 ounces	2.4 or less
Vermouth, sweet	1 ounce	2.4

Moderate Fructose

Brandy	1.5 ounces	6.8

High Fructose

Coffee liqueur	1.5 ounces	9.7
Wine cooler	12 ounces	17.6

[1] Has no fructose, but is very high in purines

SWEETENERS

SWEETENER	SERVING SIZE	GRAMS OF FRUCTOSE

Low Fructose

Powdered sugar	1 teaspoon	1.2
Table sugar	1 teaspoon	2.0

SWEETENER	SERVING SIZE	GRAMS OF FRUCTOSE
Brown sugar	1 teaspoon	2.1

Moderate Fructose

Molasses	1 tablespoon	5.5

High Fructose

Honey	1 tablespoon	8.8

DESSERTS AND DESSERT TOPPINGS

DESSERT OR TOPPING	SERVING SIZE	GRAMS OF FRUCTOSE

Fructose Free/Very Low Fructose

Canned whipped cream (light, regular, or heavy)	2 tablespoons	0.5
Nondairy whipped topping	2 tablespoons	0.5

Low Fructose

Canned whipped cream (fat free)	2 tablespoons	1.0

Moderate Fructose

Chocolate chip cookie	1	3.6
Bread pudding	½ cup	4.0
Baked custard	½ cup	5.0
Rice pudding with raisins	½ cup	5.5
Butterscotch pudding	½ cup	6.0
Pecan Danish ring coffee cake	1 slice	6.0
Sponge cake	1 slice	7.0
Coconut frosting	2 tablespoons	7.6
Whipped cream cheese frosting	2 tablespoons	7.6
Coconut macaroon	1 medium	8.0

DESSERT OR TOPPING	SERVING SIZE	GRAMS OF FRUCTOSE
High Fructose		
Ice cream	½ cup	8.2
Chocolate syrup	2 tablespoons	9.7
Éclair	1	10.0
Glazed doughnut	1	10.0
Brownie	1 medium	10.0
Chocolate mousse	½ cup	14.0
Berry cobbler	1 slice (1/10 pie)	14.4
Flan	1 serving	16.0
Peach cobbler	1 slice (1/10 pie)	16.5
Apple pie	1 slice (⅛ pie)	16.5
New York–style cheesecake	1 slice (1/10 cake)	17.6
Cherry pie	1 slice (⅛ pie)	21.0
Pecan pie	1 slice (⅛ pie)	22.0
Carrot layer cake with cream cheese frosting	1 slice (1/12 pie)	27.0
Double chocolate cake	1 slice (1/10 cake)	37.0

THE FRUCTOSE CONTENT OF POPULAR FAST FOODS

Restaurant menus are subject to change; some items may not be available at all locations.

BURGER KING

MENU ITEM	SERVING SIZE	GRAMS OF FRUCTOSE
Fructose Free/Very Low Fructose		
Chicken Tenders	6-piece serving	0
Hash brown potatoes	1 small	0
French fries	1 medium	0.1
Jalapeño poppers	4-piece serving	0.5
Low Fructose		
Croissant with sausage and cheese	1	1.2
Big Fish sandwich	1	1.3
Bacon, egg, and cheese breakfast biscuit	1	2.0
Onion rings	1 medium	2.0
Bull's-Eye barbecue sauce	1 packet	2.5
Chicken sandwich, original	1	3.0
Moderate Fructose		
Hamburger	1	3.6
French Toast Sticks	5-piece serving	4.6
Breakfast syrup	1 packet	7.0
Whopper	1	7.5

MENU ITEM	SERVING SIZE	GRAMS OF FRUCTOSE
High Fructose		
Honey dipping sauce	1 packet	8.5
Hershey's Sundae Pie	1	9.8
Mini sweet roll with vanilla icing	4 rolls	10.0
Vanilla milk shake	1 small	10.8
Chocolate milk shake	1 small	20.0
Cherry Minute Maid Frozen Dessert	1 medium	45.0
Coca-Cola Classic Frozen Dessert	1 medium	45.0

DAIRY QUEEN

MENU ITEM	SERVING SIZE	GRAMS OF FRUCTOSE
Moderate Fructose		
Vanilla soft-serve ice cream	½ cup	6.5
High Fructose		
Chocolate Dilly Bar	1	8.0
Vanilla soft-serve cone	1 small	10.5
Strawberry sundae	1 small	22.0
Cappuccino MooLatté	16 ounces	26.5
Oreo Cookies Blizzard	1 small	28.0
Chocolate Xtreme Blizzard Cake, undecorated	⅛ of 8-inch cake	32.0
Banana split	1	34.5
Chocolate shake	1 small	35.0
Brownie Earthquake	1	41.5
Chocolate malt	1 small	42.0
Reese's Peanut Butter Cup Blizzard	1 large	60.5

DOMINO'S PIZZA

MENU ITEM	SERVING SIZE	GRAMS OF FRUCTOSE
Fructose Free/Very Low Fructose		
Cheese pizza, Crunchy Thin Crust, 14 inch	1 slice	0.4
Buffalo wings	1 wing	0.6
Low Fructose		
Ultimate Deep Dish Pepperoni pizza, 14 inch	1 slice	1.1
Cinna Stix	1 piece	1.5
America's Favorite Feast pizza, hand tossed, 12 inch	2 slices	2.3
Veggie Feast pizza, hand tossed, 12 inch	2 slices	2.7
Hawaiian Feast pizza, hand tossed, 12 inch	2 slices	3.3
Bacon Barbecue Feast pizza, hand tossed, 12 inch	2 slices	4.4

KENTUCKY FRIED CHICKEN

MENU ITEM	SERVING SIZE	GRAMS OF FRUCTOSE
Fructose Free/Very Low Fructose		
Hot wings	5 wings	0
Mashed potatoes with gravy	Individual serving	0.4 or less
Low Fructose		
KFC Snacker	1	1.9 or less
Potato salad	Individual serving	2.0
Corn on the cob	1 small	2.5
Moderate Fructose		
Honey BBQ wings	5 wings	4.5
Honey BBQ KFC Snacker	1	6.0

MENU ITEM	SERVING SIZE	GRAMS OF FRUCTOSE
High Fructose		
Honey BBQ chicken sandwich	1	8.0
Cole slaw	Individual serving	8.5
Baked beans	Individual serving	10.0
Little Bucket fudge brownie	1	15.0
Little Bucket lemon crème	1	26.0

MCDONALD'S

MENU ITEM	SERVING SIZE	GRAMS OF FRUCTOSE
Fructose Free/Very Low Fructose		
Chicken McNuggets	6 pieces	0
French fries	1 small	0
Fried chicken strips	1	0
Sausage burrito	1	0.1
Sausage biscuit	1	0.4
Egg McMuffin	1	0.5
Grilled chicken club sandwich	1	0.9
Low Fructose		
Caesar salad dressing	1 packet	1.0
Hotcake	1	1.1
Filet-O-Fish sandwich	1	2.0
Caesar salad with grilled chicken	1 serving	2.6
Moderate Fructose		
Hamburger	1	3.2
Quarter Pounder hamburger	1	4.0
Big Mac with cheese	1	4.2
Barbecue sauce	1 packet	4.3

MENU ITEM	SERVING SIZE	GRAMS OF FRUCTOSE
Sweet and sour sauce	1 packet	4.5
Honey mustard salad dressing	1 packet	5.0
Honey	1 packet	5.4
Apple pie	1	6.3
McDonaldland cookies	1 package	6.8

High Fructose

Fruit & yogurt parfait with granola	1	8.5
Fruit & walnut salad, snack size with yogurt	1	9.5
Sweet roll	1	10.5
Hotcakes with margarine and syrup	1 serving	15.6
Low-fat strawberry sundae	1	17.6
Vanilla Triple Thick Shake	1	21.9
M&M McFlurry	1 regular	30.1

PIZZA HUT

MENU ITEM	SERVING SIZE	GRAMS OF FRUCTOSE

Fructose Free/Very Low Fructose

Hot wings	2 wings	0
Pepperoni Pan Pizza, 14 inch	1 slice	0.3
Cheese Pan Pizza, 14 inch	1 slice	0.4
Breadsticks	1 serving	0.9 or less

Low Fructose

Veggie Lover's Pan Pizza, 14 inch	1 slice	2.4
Marinara dipping sauce	1 serving	3.0

MENU ITEM	SERVING SIZE	GRAMS OF FRUCTOSE

High Fructose

MENU ITEM	SERVING SIZE	GRAMS OF FRUCTOSE
Spaghetti with meatballs	1 serving	8.0

SUBWAY

MENU ITEM	SERVING SIZE	GRAMS OF FRUCTOSE

Fructose Free/Very Low Fructose

Seafood and crab salad	1	0.5

Low Fructose

Deli-style roll	1	1.0
Minestrone soup	1 cup	1.0
Roasted chicken breast salad	1	1.0
Fat-free vinaigrette sauce	1½ tablespoons	1.5
Parmesan oregano bread	1, 6-inch	2.0
Tuna on Italian bread	1, 6-inch	2.0
Vegetable beef soup	1 cup	2.0
Cold Cut Trio on Italian bread	1, 6-inch	2.5
Turkey breast with ham, on Italian bread	1, 6-inch	2.5
Veggie Delite on Italian bread	1, 6-inch	2.5
Meatball on Italian bread	1, 6-inch	3.0

Moderate Fructose

Tomato bisque	1 cup	3.5
Fat-free sweet onion sauce	1½ tablespoons	4.0
Honey oat bread	1, 6-inch	4.5
Oatmeal raisin cookie	1	7.8

MENU ITEM	SERVING SIZE	GRAMS OF FRUCTOSE
Sweet onion chicken teriyaki, on white bread	1, 6-inch	7.8

High Fructose

MENU ITEM	SERVING SIZE	GRAMS OF FRUCTOSE
White chip macadamia cookie	1	8.5
Chocolate chip cookie	1	8.8
Peach Pizazz Fruizle	1 small	13
Sunrise Refresher Fruizle	1 small	14
Pineapple Delight with Banana Fruizle	1 small	16.5

TACO BELL

MENU ITEM	SERVING SIZE	GRAMS OF FRUCTOSE

Fructose Free/Very Low Fructose

Beef taco	1	0.3
Beef taco, soft	1	0.5
Taco sauce, mild	1 serving	0.5
Thick 'n' Chunky Salsa, medium	2 tablespoons	0.6

Low Fructose

Taco Supreme	1	1.0
Tostada	1	1.0
Chicken Fiesta burrito	1	1.6
Chalupa nacho cheese, chicken	1	1.8
Chicken quesadilla	1	2.0

Moderate Fructose

Taco salad with salsa and shell	1	3.8

WENDY'S

MENU ITEM	SERVING SIZE	GRAMS OF FRUCTOSE
Fructose Free/Very Low Fructose		
Chicken nuggets	5 pieces	0
French fries	1 medium	0.2
Low Fructose		
Garden salad without dressing	1 side	2.0
Baked potato with sour cream and chives	1	2.1
Baked potato with broccoli and cheese	1	2.4
Chili	1 small	2.5
Cheeseburger	1	2.6
Hamburger	1	2.9
Moderate Fructose		
Barbecue sauce	1 packet	4.0
Sweet and sour sauce	1 packet	5.5
Mandarin chicken salad without dressing	1	6.5
High Fructose		
Low-fat honey mustard salad dressing	1 packet	8.0
Oriental sesame salad dressing	1 packet	9.5

THE PURINE CONTENT
OF SELECTED FOODS

As a general rule, limit yourself to one serving of high-purine foods from each category per month. (In other words, if you have clams for dinner tonight, wait a month before eating another serving of high-purine fish or seafood.) Eat moderate-purine foods no more than once a day.

	FOODS THAT ARE MODERATELY HIGH IN PURINES	FOODS THAT ARE HIGH IN PURINES
Vegetables	Asparagus, cauliflower, green peas, mushrooms, spinach	
Meat and poultry	Most beef, pork, and lamb; beef soup and broth; pheasant	Organ meats (such as liver), meat extract, gravy; game meats, goose, mincemeat
Fish and seafood	Salmon and tuna	Anchovies, clams, herring, lobster, mackerel, mussels, oysters, sardines, scallops, shrimp*
Alcoholic beverages		Beer
Miscellaneous		Brewer's yeast supplements

*Shrimp is permitted twice per month.

REFERENCES

Bantle, J. P., S. K. Raatz, W. Thomas, and A. Georgopoulos. "Effects of Dietary Fructose on Plasma Lipids in Healthy Subjects." *American Journal of Clinical Nutrition* 72 (2000): 1128–34.

Barrera, C. M., Z. R. Ruiz, and W. P. Dunlap. "Uric Acid: A Participating Factor in the Symptoms of Hyperactivity." *Biological Psychiatry* 24 (1988): 344–47.

Beck-Nielsen, H., O. Pedersen, and H. O. Lindskov. "Impaired Cellular Insulin Binding and Insulin Sensitivity Induced by High-Fructose Feeding in Normal Subjects." *American Journal of Clinical Nutrition* 33 (1980): 273–8.

Blakely, S. R., J. Hallfrisch, S. Reiser, and E. S. Prather. "Long-Term Effects of Moderate Fructose Feeding on Glucose Tolerance Parameters in Rats." *Journal of Nutrition* 111 (1981): 307–14.

Bray, G. A., S. J. Nielsen, and B. M. Popkin. "Consumption of High-Fructose Corn Syrup in Beverages May Play a Role in the Epidemic of Obesity." *American Journal of Clinical Nutrition* 79 (2004): 537–43.

Critser, Greg. *Fat Land: How Americans Became the Fattest People in the World*. New York: First Mariner Books, 2004.

Dennison, B. A., H. L. Rockwell, and S. L. Baker. "Excess Fruit Juice Consumption by Preschool-Aged Children Is Associated with Short Stature and Obesity." *Pediatrics* 99 (1997): 15–22.

Elliott, S. S., N. L. Keim, J. S. Stern, K. Teff, and P. J. Havel. "Fructose, Weight Gain, and the Insulin Resistance Syndrome." *American Journal of Clinical Nutrition* 76 (2002): 911–22.

Gaby, A. R. "Adverse Effects of Dietary Fructose." *Alternative Medicine Review* 10 (2005): 294–306.

Gersch, M. S., W. Mu, P. Cirillo, S. Reungjui, L. Zhang, C. Roncal, Y. Y. Sautin, R. J. Johnson, T. Nakagawa. "Fructose, But Not Dextrose, Accelerates the Progression of Chronic Kidney Disease." *American Journal of Physiology—Renal Physiology* 293 (2007): F1256–61.

Hallfrisch, J., K. C. Ellwood, O. E. Michaelis, S. Reiser, T. M. O'Dorisio, and E. S. Prather. "Effects of Dietary Fructose on Plasma Glucose and Hormone Responses in Normal and Hyperinsulinemic Men." *Journal of Nutrition* 113 (1983): 1819–26.

Havel, P. J. "Dietary Fructose: Implications for Dysregulation of Energy Homeostasis and Lipid/Carbohydrate Metabolism." *Nutrition Reviews* 63 (2005): 133–57.

Israel, K. D., O. E. Michaelis, S. Reiser, and M. Keeney. "Serum Uric Acid, Inorganic Phosphorus, and Glutamic-Oxalacetic Transaminase and Blood Pressure in Carbohydrate-Sensitive Adults Consuming Three Different Levels of Sucrose." *Annals of Nutrition and Metabolism* 27 (1983): 425–35.

Johnson, R. J., D. H. Kang, D. Feig, S. Kivlighn, J. Kanellis, S. Watanabe, K. R. Tuttle, B. Rodriguez-Iturbe, J. Herrera-Acosta, and M. Mazzali. "Is There a Pathogenetic Role for Uric Acid in Hypertension and Cardiovascular and Renal Disease?" *Hypertension* 41 (2003): 1183–90.

Johnson, R. J., M. Segal, Y. Sautin, T. Nakagawa, D. I. Feig, D. H. Kang, M. S. Gersch, S. Benner, and L. G. Sanchez-Lozada. "Potential Role of Sugar (Fructose) in the Epidemic of Hypertension, Obesity and the Metabolic Syndrome, Diabetes, Kidney Disease, and Cardiovascular Disease." *American Journal of Clinical Nutrition* 86 (2007): 899–906.

Jurgens, H., W. Haass, T. R. Castaneda, A. Schurmann, C. Koebnick, F. Dombrowski, B. Otto, A. R. Nawrocki, P. E. Scherer, J. Spranger, M. Ristow, H. G. Joost, P. J. Havel, and M. H. Tschop. "Consuming Fructose-Sweetened Beverages Increases Body Adiposity in Mice." *Obesity Research* 13 (2005): 1146–56.

Le, K. A. and L. Tappy. "Metabolic Effects of Fructose." *Current Opinion in Clinical Nutrition and Metabolic Care* 9 (2006): 469–75.

Ludwig, D. S., K. E. Peterson, and S. L. Gortmaker. "Relation between Consumption of Sugar-Sweetened Drinks and Childhood Obesity: A Prospective, Observational Analysis." *Lancet* 357 (2001): 505–8.

Masuo, K., H. Kawaguchi, H. Mikami, T. Ogihara, and M. L. Tuck. "Serum Uric Acid and Plasma Norepinephrine Concentrations Predict Subsequent Weight Gain and Blood Pressure Elevation." *Hypertension* 42 (2003): 474–80.

Mazzali, M., J. Hughes, Y. G. Kim, J. A. Jefferson, D. H. Kang, K. L. Gordon, H. Y. Lan, S. Kivlighn, and R. J. Johnson. "Elevated Uric Acid Increases Blood Pressure in the Rat by a Novel Crystal-Independent Mechanism." *Hypertension* 38 (2001): 1101–6.

McGee, Harold. *On Food and Cooking: The Science and Lore of the Kitchen.* New York: Scribner, 2004.

Mintz, Sidney W. *Sweetness and Power: The Place of Sugar in Modern History.* New York: Penguin Books, 1986.

Nakagawa, T., H. Hu, S. Zharikov, K. R. Tuttle, R. A. Short, O. Glushakova, X. Ouyang, D. I. Feig, E. R. Block, J. Herrera-Acosta, J. M. Patel, and R. J. Johnson. "A Causal Role for Uric Acid in Fructose-Induced Metabolic Syndrome." *American Journal of Physiology—Renal Physiology* 290(3) (2006): F625–31.

Nakagawa, T. T., K. R. Tuttle, R. A. Short, and R. J. Johnson. "Fructose-Induced Hyperuricemia as a Causal Mechanism for the Epidemic of the Metabolic Syndrome." *Nature Clinical Practice Nephrology* 1 (2006): 80–86.

Nielsen, S. J. and B. M. Popkin. "Changes in Beverage Intake between 1977 and 2001." *American Journal of Preventive Medicine* 27 (2004): 205–10.

Pollan, Michael. *The Botany of Desire: A Plant's-Eye View of the World.* New York: Random House, 2001.

Porter, R., and G. S. Rousseau. *Gout: The Patrician Malady*. New Haven: Yale University Press, 2000.

Raben, A., I. Macdonald, and A. Astrup. "Replacement of Dietary Fat by Sucrose or Starch: Effects on 14 Day Ad Libitum Energy Intake, Energy Expenditure, and Body Weight in Formerly Obese and Never-Obese Subjects." *International Journal of Obesity and Related Metabolic Disorders* 21 (1997): 846–59.

Reungjui, S., C. A. Roncal, W. Mu, T. R. Srinivas, D. Sirivongs, R. J. Johnson, and T. Nakagawa. "Thiazide Diuretics Exacerbate Fructose-Induced Metabolic Syndrome." *Journal of the American Society of Nephrology* 18 (2007): 2724–31.

Sanchez-Lozada, L. G., E. Tapia, A. Jimenez, P. Bautista, M. Cristobal, T. Nepomuceno, V. Soto, C. Avila-Casado, T. Nakagawa, R. J. Johnson, J. Herrera-Acosta, and M. Franco. "Fructose-Induced Metabolic Syndrome Is Associated with Glomerular Hypertension and Renal Microvascular Damage in Rats." *American Journal of Physiology—Renal Physiology* 292 (2007): F423–9.

Schretlen, D. J., A. B. Inscore, T. D. Vannorsdall, M. Kraut, G. D. Pearlson, B. Gordon, and H. A. Jinnah. "Serum Uric Acid and Brain Ischemia in Normal Elderly Adults." *Neurology* 69 (2007): 1418–23.

Schulze, M. B., J. E. Manson, D. S. Ludwig, G. A. Colditz, M. J. Stampfer, W. C. Willett, and F. B. Hu. "Sugar-Sweetened Beverages, Weight Gain, and Incidence of Type 2 Diabetes in Young and Middle-Aged Women." *JAMA* 292 (2004): 927–34.

Segal, M. S., E. Gollub, and R. J. Johnson. "Is the Fructose Index More Relevant with Regards to Cardiovascular Disease Than the Glycemic Index?" *European Journal of Nutrition* 46 (2007); 406–17.

Stirpe, F., E. Della Corte, E. Bonetti, A. Abbondanza, A. Abbati, and F. De Stefano. "Fructose-Induced Hyperuricaemia." *Lancet* 2 (1970): 1310–1.

Teff, K. L., S. S. Elliott, M. Tschop, T. J. Kieffer, D. Rader, M. Heiman, R. R. Townsend, N. L. Keim, D. D'Alessio, and P. J. Havel. "Dietary Fructose Reduces Circulating Insulin and

Leptin, Attenuates Postprandial Suppression of Ghrelin, and Increases Triglycerides in Women." *Journal of Clinical Endocrinology and Metabolism* 89 (2004): 2963–72.

Welsh, J. A., M. E. Cogswell, S. Rogers, H. Rockett, Z. Mei, and L. M. Grummer-Strawn. "Overweight among Low-Income Preschool Children Associated with the Consumption of Sweet Drinks: Missouri, 1999–2002." *Pediatrics* 115 (2005): e223–9.

Yudkin, J. "Evolutionary and Historical Changes in Dietary Carbohydrates." *American Journal of Clinical Nutrition* 20 (1967): 108–15.

Yudkin, John. *Sweet and Dangerous*. New York: Bantam Books, 1979.

INDEX

Italic page references indicate boxed text and tables.

P

Pancreatic cancer, 138, 140
Parkinson's disease, 283
Partially hydrogenated oil, 174,
175
Pasta
Bowtie Pasta Salad, 312–13
Grilled Chicken Breasts over
Orzo Pasta with Artichoke
Hearts and Feta Cheese,
329–30
in Low-Fructose Diet, 169
Marvelous and Meatless,
310–11
Neapolitan Casserole,
314–15
recommended consumption of,
239–40
Phenylketonuria, 180
Polyunsaturated fats, 174
Potassium-rich foods, 252–53
Potassium supplements, 252,
260, 261
Potatoes, *167*
Poultry. *See also* Chicken
purines in, *370*
recommended consumption of,
171, 239
Preeclampsia, fructose and,
141
Pregnancy, *141*, 180, *265*
Prehypertension, 182
Probenecid, 255
Prostate cancer, fructose and,
139
Pudding
Rice Pudding, 346–47
Purines
in alcoholic beverages, *80*, 81,
184, 241, *370*
avoiding, in Fructose-Free
Phase, 206, 211–12
definition of, 78

in fish and shellfish, 81,
171–72, 237, 239, *370*
in legumes, 168
limiting consumption of, 237,
370
in meats, 170–71, 238–39,
370
in organ meats, 81, 170–71,
238–39, *370*
in vegetables, 81, 167–68,
237–38, *370*

R

Rectal cancer, 139
Restaurant foods, Fructose-Free
Phase and, 212
Resveratrol, heart protection
from, 185
Rice, 168–69, 239–40
Rice Pudding, 346–47

S

Saccharin, 179, 212
Salad dressings, fructose content
of, *356*
Salt, 181–83, 217, 240
Saturated fat, 174, 240
Shellfish. *See* Fish and shellfish
Short stature, from fruit juice,
137
Skin cancer, 249
Sodium. *See* Salt
Soft drinks
consumption of, 24, 31–34
fountain, fructose content of,
33
HFCS in, 28, 31–32, 40, 127,
176, *177*
history of, 24
milk consumption replaced by,
187
NAFLD and, 134, *134*